WORKBOOK

HIGH RELIABILITY ORGANIZATIONS
THIRD EDITION

A Healthcare Handbook for Patient Safety & Quality

CYNTHIA A. OSTER, PhD, MBA, APRN, ACNS-BC, CNS-BC, ANP, FAAN
JANE S. BRAATEN, PhD, APRN, CNS, ANP, CPPS, CPHQ

Contributors:
Noreen Bernard, EdD, RN, NEA-BC, FAAN
Kristen A. Oster, DNP, EMBA, APRN, ACNS-BC, CNOR, CNS-CP

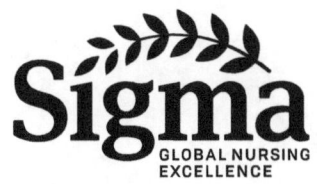

Copyright © 2026 by Sigma Theta Tau International Honor Society of Nursing

All rights reserved. This book is protected by copyright. No part of it may be reproduced, stored in a retrieval system, or transmitted in any form or by any means, electronic, mechanical, photocopying, recording, or otherwise, without written permission from the publisher. Any trademarks, service marks, design rights, or similar rights that are mentioned, used, or cited in this book are the property of their respective owners. Their use here does not imply that you may use them for a similar or any other purpose.

This book is not intended to be a substitute for the medical advice of a licensed medical professional. The author and publisher have made every effort to ensure the accuracy of the information contained within at the time of its publication and shall have no liability or responsibility to any person or entity regarding any loss or damage incurred, or alleged to have incurred, directly or indirectly, by the information contained in this book. The author and publisher make no warranties, express or implied, with respect to its content, and no warranties may be created or extended by sales representatives or written sales materials. The author and publisher have no responsibility for the consistency or accuracy of URLs and content of third-party websites referenced in this book.

Sigma Theta Tau International Honor Society of Nursing (Sigma) is a nonprofit organization whose mission is advancing world health and celebrating nursing excellence in scholarship, leadership, and service. Founded in 1922, Sigma has more than 90,000 active members in over 100 countries and territories. Members include practicing nurses, instructors, researchers, policymakers, entrepreneurs, and others. Sigma's more than 540 chapters are located at more than 700 institutions of higher education throughout Armenia, Australia, Botswana, Brazil, Canada, Colombia, England, Eswatini, Ghana, Hong Kong, Ireland, Israel, Jamaica, Japan, Jordan, Kenya, Lebanon, Malawi, Mexico, the Netherlands, Nigeria, Pakistan, Philippines, Portugal, Puerto Rico, Scotland, Singapore, South Africa, South Korea, Sweden, Taiwan, Tanzania, Thailand, the United States, and Wales. Learn more at www.sigmanursing.org.

Sigma Theta Tau International
550 West North Street
Indianapolis, IN, USA 46202

To request a review copy for course adoption, order additional books, buy in bulk, or purchase for corporate use, contact Sigma Marketplace at 888.654.4968 (US/Canada toll-free), +1.317.687.2256 (International), or solutions@sigmamarketplace.org.

To request author information, or for speaker or other media requests, contact Sigma Marketing at 888.634.7575 (US/Canada toll-free) or +1.317.634.8171 (International).

ISBN: 9781646481897
ISBN EPUB: 9781646481590
ISBN PDF: 9781646481583

Publisher: Dustin Sullivan
Acquisitions Editor: Emily Hatch
Development Editor: Jillmarie Leeper Sycamore
Cover Designer: Michael Tanamachi
Interior Design/Page Layout: Rebecca Batchelor

Managing Editor: Carla Hall
Project Editor: Todd Lothery
Copy Editor: Todd Lothery
Proofreader: Todd Lothery

ACKNOWLEDGMENTS

The authors wish to thank Noreen Bernard and Kristen Oster for contributing their expertise and clinical experiences to make this workbook relevant to both facilitator and student.

Special thanks to Jennifer Kimberlain, MSN, RN, MBA-HA, CPPS, for providing valuable feedback to the content of the workbook.

ABOUT THE EDITORS

Cynthia A. Oster, PhD, MBA, APRN, ACNS-BC, CNS-BC, ANP, FAAN, is the Enterprise Nurse Scientist – Research Program Manager for the Mountain Region of CommonSpirit Health in Centennial, Colorado, following four years of service as the Patient Safety Nurse Scientist at Emory Healthcare and adjunct Assistant Professor at the Nell Hodgson Woodruff School of Nursing at Emory University in Atlanta, Georgia. For more than a decade, Oster was a nurse scientist for Centura Health and a clinical nurse specialist for critical care and cardiovascular services at AdventHealth Porter in Denver, Colorado. She has held research, clinical, educational, and administrative positions throughout her more than 40-year career. Oster received her BSN from the University of Iowa, her MSN from the University of Nebraska Medical Center, and her PhD from the University of Colorado College of Nursing. In addition, she earned an ANP certificate from Beth El College of Nursing in Colorado Springs, Colorado, and an MBA from the University of Colorado–Denver. She holds Clinical Nurse Specialist-Core and Adult Clinical Nurse Specialist certification from the American Nurses Credentialing Center. In 2017, she became a Fellow in the American Academy of Nursing. She mentors clinical nurses and advanced practice nurses to develop clinical practice wisdom through application of high reliability principles, evidence-based practice, and the conduct of research. Oster has presented at national and international meetings and has published in the areas of high reliability, evidence-based practice, alarm fatigue, and peer review. She is a member of Sigma Theta Tau International, the American Nurses Association, the American Association of Critical-Care Nurses, the National Association of Clinical Nurse Specialists, the American College of Healthcare Executives, and Beta Gamma Sigma.

Jane S. Braaten, PhD, APRN, CNS, ANP, CPPS, CPHQ, is a Regional Director of Patient Safety and High Reliability at Commonspirit Health® in Centennial, Colorado. She has held positions as Director of Cardiology Services, Cardiac and Intensive Care Clinical Nurse Specialist, Cardiac Nurse Practitioner, and Manager/Charge RN/Staff RN of intensive care and telemetry units. Braaten obtained her BSN from the Indiana University School of Nursing and holds the degree of doctor of philosophy, a master's degree as a clinical nurse specialist, and a certificate as an adult nurse practitioner from the University of Colorado College of Nursing. She also is a certified professional in patient safety (CPPS) and a certified professional in healthcare quality (CPHQ). She has presented at national meetings and has published in the areas of hospital system barriers to rapid response team activation, quality improvement in telemetry, end-of-life care in the intensive care unit, leadership, and high reliability organizations and healthcare. She is a passionate mentor and supporter to those at the front line who create safe patient care daily.

ABOUT THE CONTRIBUTORS

Noreen Bernard, EdD, RN, NEA-BC, FAAN, is a distinguished nurse executive with extensive experience in shaping nursing practice across both acute care and ambulatory settings. As a Chief Nursing Officer overseeing multiple sites within a prominent health system, Bernard excels in executive systems leadership, clinical operations, and workforce strategies, driving nursing excellence and enhancing professional practice. Her commitment to high reliability is reflected in her focus on improving quality and patient safety outcomes. In addition to her executive role, Bernard contributes to academia as an adjunct faculty member and doctoral program content expert at two universities. Her scholarly work spans several critical areas, including nursing administration, resilience, job satisfaction, professional joy, leader development, and nursing practice. Bernard is also actively involved in the academic community as a volunteer editor and board member for three national journals. Bernard earned her doctor of education in organizational leadership and organization development from Grand Canyon University, her master's in nursing administration from the University of Colorado, and her BSN from the University of Northern Colorado. She is Nurse Executive Advanced Board Certified and was honored as a Fellow in the American Academy of Nursing in 2019. Her professional journey reflects a steadfast dedication to advancing the field of nursing through leadership, research, and education.

Kristen A. Oster, DNP, EMBA, APRN, ACNS-BC, CNOR, CNS-CP, is currently the Director of Surgical Services at Intermountain Health Good Samaritan Hospital in Lafayette, Colorado. She has held a variety of perioperative and ambulatory positions throughout her career, including operating room and pain procedural care clinical manager; assistant nurse manager for an ENT, skull base, head/neck, and neurosurgery service line; perioperative clinical nurse specialist; clinical manager for geographic float pools; and regional nursing services coordinator supporting ambulatory services. She was the Patient Safety Specialist assigned to the perioperative and ambulatory service line at the University of Colorado–Anschutz Medical Campus in Aurora, Colorado. She received a bachelor of science degree in biology and education from Denison University in Granville, Ohio. Oster earned a bachelor of science degree in nursing from the accelerated nursing program at Regis University, Denver, Colorado. She holds a master of science in nursing degree—clinical nurse specialist focus in adult and geriatric acute care and Doctorate in Nursing Practice—from the University of Colorado, Denver. She completed her executive master's in business administration at the University of Colorado, Denver. Oster is a member of the Association of periOperative Registered Nurses and American Organization of Nursing Leadership.

TABLE OF CONTENTS

About the Editors iv
About the Contributors v
Introduction x

PART I   HIGH RELIABILITY: THE IMPERATIVE REMAINS 1

1   HIGH RELIABILITY: REFLECTIONS ON THE ESSENCE OF HRO AND THE APPLICATION TO HEALTHCARE 2

Learning Activity 1.1: Compare and Contrast External/Internal Drivers Shaping the Healthcare Quality and Safety Paradigm Shift 3

2   DRIVERS FOR PATIENT SAFETY 5

Learning Activity 2.1: Differentiate Individual and System Factors Within Patient Harm Events Through Application of High Reliability Principles to Discover Solutions and Explore Barriers 6

3   CURRENT QUALITY DRIVERS 8

Learning Activity 3.1: Discover How Evidence-Based Practice Aligns With High Reliability Principles to Inform Drivers of Quality 9

4   ORGANIZATIONAL CULTURE AND PSYCHOLOGICAL SAFETY: BREAKING DOWN BARRIERS 11

Learning Activity 4.1: Compare and Contrast Facilitators and Barriers of Psychological Safety and Discuss Practical Measures of Psychological Safety 12

5   SAFETY LEADERSHIP: COMMITMENT TO HIGH RELIABILITY ORGANIZING ... 14

Learning Activity 5.1: Compare and Contrast Characteristics of Safety Leadership Styles and Safety Leadership Actions Within a High Reliability Organizing Framework 15

6   HEALTH EQUITY AND HIGH RELIABILITY: CONNECTING THE DOTS FOR PATIENT SAFETY 20

Learning Activity 6.1: Use Health Equity Knowledge to Inform Patient Safety Initiatives 21

PART II   HRO CONCEPTS AND APPLICATION TO PRACTICE: PREOCCUPATION WITH FAILURE 24

7   USING FAILURE MODE AND EFFECTS ANALYSIS TO PREDICT FAILURE 25

Learning Activity 7.1: Discuss the Importance of the FMEA Process Within a High Reliability Organization 26

8   PAYING ATTENTION TO CLOSE CALLS AND NEAR MISSES 29

Learning Activity 8.1: Evaluate the Importance of Near Misses, Close Calls, and Unsafe Conditions to High Reliability 30

PART III HRO CONCEPTS AND APPLICATION TO PRACTICE: RELUCTANCE TO SIMPLIFY 32

9 HUMAN FACTORS ENGINEERING FOR REDUCING AND RECOVERING ERROR ... 33

Learning Activity 9.1: Explain Human Factors Engineering (HFE): The Science and Practice of Designing Work Systems to Fit the Needs, Limitations, and Capabilities of Humans 34

10 ROOT CAUSE ANALYSIS: A TOOL FOR HIGH RELIABILITY IN A COMPLEX ENVIRONMENT 36

Learning Activity 10.1: Discuss Use of RCA as a Tool for Embedding the High Reliability Principle "Reluctance to Simplify" Into a Safety Event Investigation 37

11 FOSTERING JUST CULTURE IN HIGH RELIABILITY ORGANIZATIONS: HOW FAR HAVE WE COME? 39

Learning Activity 11.1: Examine the Features and Challenges of a Just Culture Within a Highly Reliable Safety Program and the Current Healthcare Environment 40

PART IV HRO CONCEPTS AND APPLICATION TO PRACTICE: SENSITIVITY TO OPERATIONS 43

12 ALARM SAFETY: WORKING SOLUTIONS 44

Learning Activity 12.1: Appraise the Concept of Alarm Fatigue and the Possibilities for Improvement When Applying High Reliability Principles to Clinical Alarm Safety 45

13 INNOVATIVE TECHNOLOGY, STANDARDIZATION, AND THE IMPACT ON HIGH RELIABILITY 47

Learning Activity 13.1: Apply Knowledge of Effective Interventions for High Reliability to Analyze Technological Advances in Your Practice 48

14 TIERED SAFETY HUDDLES 51

Learning Activity 14.1: Describe the Value of the Tiered Huddle in Healthcare as an Effective Tool to Promote High Reliability in a Complex Organization 52

PART V HRO CONCEPTS AND APPLICATION TO PRACTICE: DEFERENCE TO EXPERTISE 54

15 THE CURRENT NEED FOR INTERPROFESSIONAL COLLABORATIVE CARE AND TEAMWORK 55

Learning Activity 15.1: Describe and Explain an Interprofessional Team in the Context of HROs ... 56

16 MEANINGFUL PATIENT ENGAGEMENT: BEST PRACTICE FOR HIGH RELIABILITY 58

Learning Activity 16.1: Explain Meaningful Patient and Family Engagement in the Context of High Reliability for Patient Safety and Quality 59

17 PEDIATRIC PATIENT SAFETY: UTILIZING SAFETY COACHING AS A STRATEGY TOWARD ZERO HARM 61

Learning Activity 17.1: Examine the Role of Safety Coaches as a Vehicle for Successful Change Management and Sustainability of HRO Principles 62

PART VI HRO CONCEPTS AND APPLICATION TO PRACTICE: COMMITMENT TO RESILIENCE 65

18 DESIGNING RESILIENCE INTO THE WORK ENVIRONMENT 66

Learning Activity 18.1: Apply a Social-Ecological Perspective of Resilience to Support Clinician Well-Being in the Work Environment 67

19 BUILDING HIGH RELIABILITY THROUGH SIMULATION 69

Learning Activity 19.1: Explore Opportunities to Use Simulation to Improve Safety and Reliability of Risk-Prone Processes 70

20 BUILDING RESILIENCE THROUGH TEAM TRAINING: RAPID RESPONSE AND IN-HOSPITAL CARDIAC ARREST EVENTS 71

Learning Activity 20.1: Evaluate Rapid Response and In-Hospital Cardiac Arrest Event Team Performance 72

21 SUSTAINING A CULTURE OF SAFETY 75

Learning Activity 21.1: Focus on Sustaining a Culture of Safety in a Resilient Organization 76

PART VII ASSIMILATION INTO PRACTICE ACROSS THE CONTINUUM 78

22 AMBULATORY CARE: THE FRONTIER FOR HIGH RELIABILITY 79

Learning Activity 22.1: Integrate High Reliability Principles to Address Quality and Safety Challenges in Ambulatory Care 80

23 THE SYNTHESIS AMONG MAGNET RECOGNITION PROGRAM® MODEL COMPONENTS AND HIGH RELIABILITY ORGANIZATION PRINCIPLES 81

Learning Activity 23.1: Explain the Synergistic Relationship Between the Magnet Model Components and the Principles of High Reliability 82

24 REALIZING HIGH RELIABILITY: NURSE SCIENTIST AND BEDSIDE SCIENTIST COLLABORATION 84

Learning Activity 24.1: Discover the Role of the Nurse Scientist and Bedside Scientist in a High Reliability Organization 85

25 ENSURING HIGH RELIABILITY IN ACUTE STROKE TREATMENT 87

Learning Activity 25.1: Apply High Reliability Principles to Acute Stroke Treatment 88

PART VIII TRANSLATION INTO PRACTICE 89

26 HIGH RELIABILITY PERFORMANCE DURING A PANDEMIC 90
Learning Activity 26.1: Explore High Reliability Performance During a Pandemic 91

27 BUILDING A HIGH RELIABILITY HEAD AND NECK OPERATING ROOM TEAM 92
Learning Activity 27.1: Apply High Reliability Principles to Solve Team Quality and Safety Challenges 93

28 DECREASING HARM FROM WORKPLACE VIOLENCE 96
Learning Activity 28.1: Discuss Causes, Consequences, and Interventions to Workplace Violence in Healthcare 97

29 INTRODUCTION OF HIGH RELIABILITY TO FRONTLINE STAFF: CREATING A VIRTUAL RESOURCE TOOLKIT 99
Learning Activity 29.1: Apply High Reliability Principles to Solve Organizational Team Quality and Safety Challenges 100

PART IX TRANSLATION INTO PRACTICE SUMMATIVE ASSESSMENT 103

SUMMATIVE ASSESSMENT: TRANSLATION INTO PRACTICE 104
Summative Assessment Learning Activity: Translate Evidence-Based Practice, Change Management, and High Reliability Principles to Practice 105

SUPPLEMENTAL RESOURCES AND READINGS 107

INTRODUCTION

ABOUT THE WORKBOOK

As a student in a healthcare profession, you have probably heard of the concept of *high reliability* as a means to reduce harm, enhance quality, and improve outcomes. Patient safety and quality are of increasing importance to consumers, payers, providers, and organizations. The quest for high reliability must permeate an organization by way of leadership commitment, a culture of safety, continuous quality improvement, and every person's focus within the organization. This workbook is designed as a companion to the primary textbook, *High Reliability Organizations: A Healthcare Handbook for Patient Safety & Quality* (3rd ed.), which explains how high reliability contributes to organizational quality and safety, recommends quality and safety activities based on high reliability principles, and integrates high reliability principles into healthcare practice.

PURPOSE AND STRUCTURE

The purpose of the *Workbook for High Reliability Organizations* (3rd ed.) is to provide learning activities that relate to each chapter in the book. These learning activities introduce you to high reliability, explain the concepts of high reliability and high reliability organizations (HROs), provide examples of what the concepts would look like in everyday practice, and describe the information and tools nurses and other healthcare providers need for the organization to become an HRO. A summative course assessment or final learning activity is also included.

Every learning activity reflects the content of its accompanying chapter. You should read the chapter and supplemental materials and, if specified, focus on certain sections within the chapter prior to completing an exercise. You may complete all these learning activities, but some facilitators may choose only one or two from each chapter that meet the objectives of a particular course. Each learning activity begins with objectives, contains accompanying resource material or additional external resources, and has learning activity exercise-specific instructions.

Nurses represent the majority of healthcare workers and are on the front lines of delivery and provision of safe and effective care. As a result, nurses are ideally situated to drive the mission to achieve high reliability in healthcare. It is our hope that this workbook will prepare you to apply HRO principles to patient safety and quality problems in your place of practice because we all benefit from a safer healthcare environment.

PART I

HIGH RELIABILITY: THE IMPERATIVE REMAINS

Learning Objective

Explain how high reliability contributes to organizational quality and safety (*analyzing*).

Contents

Chapter 1 High Reliability: Reflections on the Essence of HRO and the Application to Healthcare 2

Chapter 2 Drivers for Patient Safety 5

Chapter 3 Current Quality Drivers 8

Chapter 4 Organizational Culture and Psychological Safety: Breaking Down Barriers 11

Chapter 5 Safety Leadership: Commitment to High Reliability Organizing 14

Chapter 6 Health Equity and High Reliability: Connecting the Dots for Patient Safety 20

CHAPTER 1

HIGH RELIABILITY: REFLECTIONS ON THE ESSENCE OF HRO AND THE APPLICATION TO HEALTHCARE

In this chapter, you will learn about how high reliability has evolved over the years and the challenges still facing healthcare as we strive to create highly reliable environments.

Learning Objective

Discuss the depth of the message of high reliability and the contributors essential to creating a successful HRO environment.

Learning Activity 1.1: Compare and Contrast External/Internal Drivers Shaping the Healthcare Quality and Safety Paradigm Shift

Learning Activity Objectives

1.1 Compare external and internal drivers of quality and safety in the current healthcare system (*analyzing*).

1.2 Discuss high reliability and barriers to successful application (*understanding*).

1.3 Explain a current application of high reliability that has produced relevant safety outcomes (*applying*).

Preparation

Prior to completion of the learning activity, you should:

- Read Chapter 1.
- Read "High Reliability Organizing in Healthcare: Still a Long Way Left to Go" at https://doi.org/10.1136/bmjqs-2021-014141.

Instructions

1.1 Using Table 1.1, identify internal and external drivers in healthcare. Include how these drivers affect quality and patient safety at both the system and the unit level.

TABLE 1.1 INTERNAL AND EXTERNAL DRIVERS IN HEALTHCARE

External Drivers	Definition	Example	Macro Impact on Healthcare System	Micro Impact on Healthcare Facility (unit)

continues

TABLE 1.1 INTERNAL AND EXTERNAL DRIVERS IN HEALTHCARE (CONT.)

Internal Drivers	Definition	Example	Macro Impact on Healthcare System	Micro Impact on Healthcare Facility

1.2 Compare and contrast how application of high reliability varies in understanding. Discuss an "artifact" of high reliability in your organization and how it encourages high reliability thinking.

_____

_____

_____

_____

1.3 Present an article from the literature using at least one principle of high reliability in a healthcare setting. Include the following in the discussion: Identify the high reliability principle, define the high reliability principle, and explain how the high reliability principle was applied in the article.

_____

_____

_____

_____

CHAPTER 2

DRIVERS FOR PATIENT SAFETY

In this chapter, you will learn about the drivers for patient safety within the context of high reliability principles to better understand patient harm and its impact. You will also learn about drivers for patient safety that relate to the individual and to shared accountability across the system of care.

Learning Objective

Summarize safety drivers affecting healthcare delivery systems and explore how HROs contribute to patient safety.

Learning Activity 2.1: Differentiate Individual and System Factors Within Patient Harm Events Through Application of High Reliability Principles to Discover Solutions and Explore Barriers

Learning Activity Objectives

2.1 Describe the multiple layers and perspectives of patient harm in an HRO (*understanding*).

2.2 Explain the interconnection of high reliability and safety culture (*applying*).

2.3 Appraise current solutions for improving safety in HROs (*analyzing*).

2.4 Consider historical and current barriers to highly reliable solutions (*evaluating*).

Preparation

Prior to completion of the learning activity, you should:

- Read Chapter 2.
- View the video *The Josie King Story* at https://www.youtube.com/watch?v=xA22_QEWapo. Consider individual and system factors that led to the error.
- Read "Human Error: Models and Management" at https://doi.org/10.1136/bmj.320.7237.768.

Instructions

2.1 Define and give two examples of latent and active failures that lead to patient harm, using Table 2.1 to record your answers.

TABLE 2.1 LATENT AND ACTIVE FAILURES

	Definition	Examples From Your Experience
Latent failures (blunt end)		
Active failures (sharp end)		

2.2 Describe the Swiss cheese model of error.
- Discuss the latent factors and how they may contribute to error.
- Discuss the impact of strong and weak barriers that allow or prevent harm.
- Discuss system controls and individual controls that might strengthen barriers (block the holes in the Swiss cheese).

_____
_____
_____
_____
_____
_____
_____

2.3 Find two definitions of a safety culture: Discuss solutions and barriers to achieving a safety culture based on the definitions in your current context.
- Discuss two individual factors as antidotes to patient harm.
- Discuss two system factors as antidotes to patient harm.

_____
_____
_____
_____
_____
_____

2.4 Present an adverse event (from experience or the literature) that led to harm.
- Apply one principle of high reliability that might have prevented the outcome.
- Discuss barriers to the principle identified.

_____
_____
_____
_____
_____

CHAPTER 3

CURRENT QUALITY DRIVERS

In this chapter, you will learn about current quality drivers for patient and healthcare outcomes. You will also learn about high reliability as a framework for developing and sustaining a culture within healthcare organizations to provide care that minimizes errors and embraces current best evidence to achieve exceptional performance in quality, safety, and cost effectiveness.

Learning Objective

Explain current evidence-based quality drivers in the context of high reliability.

Learning Activity 3.1: Discover How Evidence-Based Practice Aligns With High Reliability Principles to Inform Drivers of Quality

Learning Activity Objectives

3.1 Describe four key drivers of current quality indicators (*remembering*).

3.2 Discuss the interrelationships between the drivers (*understanding*).

3.3 Identify two key quality nursing indicators and improvement ideas based on high reliability principles (*applying*).

Preparation

Prior to completion of the learning activity, you should:

- Read Chapter 3.
- Read "Deimplementation in Clinical Practice. What Are We Waiting For?" at https://doi.org/10.4037/aacnacc2019607.
- Read "Building Cultures of High Reliability: Lessons From the High Reliability Organization Paradigm" at https://doi.org/10.1016/j.anclin.2023.03.012.

Instructions

3.1 Select an evidence-based practice (EBP) model from the literature or your organization. Using Table 3.1, provide a short rationale for model selection and a brief overview.

TABLE 3.1 EVIDENCE-BASED PRACTICE MODEL

Evidence-Based Practice Model: Rationale for Selection: Brief Overview:				
Key Focus/Emphasis	**Key Concepts**	**Steps/Stages**	**Strengths**	**Limitations**

3.2 Identify one Nursing Quality Indicator and one Hospital Consumer Assessment of Healthcare Providers and Systems (HCAHPS) item. Using Table 3.2, include evidence from the literature supporting the quality indicator and HCAHPS item and a national benchmark for each.

TABLE 3.2 NURSING QUALITY INDICATOR AND HCAHPS

Nursing Quality Indicator:

Indicator Definition/Description	Supporting Evidence/Sources	National Benchmark/Benchmark Source

HCAHPS Item:

Item Definition/Description	Supporting Evidence/Sources	National Benchmark/Benchmark Source

3.3 Apply the steps of an EBP model aligned with principles of high reliability to change practice, using Table 3.3 to record your answers.

TABLE 3.3 EBP MODEL AND HIGH RELIABILITY

EBP Model:

Steps	High Reliability Principle Alignment

CHAPTER 4

ORGANIZATIONAL CULTURE AND PSYCHOLOGICAL SAFETY: BREAKING DOWN BARRIERS

In this chapter, you will learn about organizational and safety culture. You will also learn about the cultural component of psychological safety and the importance of leadership and leader actions in developing psychological safety.

Learning Objective

Examine psychological safety as a cultural component of organizational and safety culture.

Learning Activity 4.1: Compare and Contrast Facilitators and Barriers of Psychological Safety and Discuss Practical Measures of Psychological Safety

Learning Activity Objectives

4.1 Compare characteristics of a psychologically and non-psychologically safe workplace (*understanding*).

4.2 Show facilitators and barriers to psychological safety (*understanding*).

4.3 Illustrate how an organization measures psychological safety in a high reliability culture of safety (*understanding*).

Preparation

Prior to completion of the learning activity, you should:

- Read Chapter 4.
- Read "Defining and Assessing Organizational Culture" at https://doi.org/10.1111/j.1744-6198.2010.00207.x.
- Read "What Is Psychological Safety?" at https://hbr.org/2023/02/what-is-psychological-safety.

Instructions

4.1 Define and observe deep-seated assumptions and beliefs, espoused values, and artifacts of culture within your own organization.

Assumptions and beliefs: What are the driving forces behind your organization? This could be religious affiliation, for profit, not for profit, and so on. These assumptions and beliefs may be hidden, but they drive the values and artifacts of your culture.

My organization believes that . . . .

_____

_____

_____

Espoused values: What is the written vision or mission statement of your organization?

Our vision or mission statement is written as . . .

_____

_____

_____

Artifacts: The visible manifestations of the values and beliefs of the system. This can include policies, art in the hospital, work environment, standard behaviors, expectations of leaders, reward systems, and more.

Our values are made visible by . . .

_____

_____

_____

4.2 Discuss characteristics of psychological safety and non-psychological safety in the workplace using Table 4.1. Include facilitators and barriers.

TABLE 4.1 PSYCHOLOGICAL SAFETY IN THE WORKPLACE

Psychologically Safe Environment				
Event	What Happens at Your Organization?	Psychologically or Non-Psychologically Safe Workplace?	Facilitator	Barrier
Non- Psychologically Safe Environment				
Event	What Happens at Your Organization?	Psychologically or Non-Psychologically Safe Workplace?	Facilitator	Barrier

4.3 Illustrate how an organization measures psychological safety in a high reliability culture of safety in an online discussion.

- Does the organization measure psychological safety?
- Describe the measurement instrument and why it was selected.
- What are the current measures of psychological safety?
- What is the best and lowest performing category?
- How would you go about improving the scores?
- What facilitators and barriers do you see to improving scores?

CHAPTER 5

SAFETY LEADERSHIP: COMMITMENT TO HIGH RELIABILITY ORGANIZING

In this chapter, you will learn about the vital role of leadership in creating an HRO. You will also learn about safety leadership style and associated safety leadership actions in a high reliability organizing framework to create the fearless workplace.

Learning Objective

Explain and discuss the vital role of leadership in an HRO.

Learning Activity 5.1: Compare and Contrast Characteristics of Safety Leadership Styles and Safety Leadership Actions Within a High Reliability Organizing Framework

Learning Activity Objectives

5.1 Describe the influence of different safety leadership styles and safety leadership actions on high reliability organizational quality and safety (*understanding*).

5.2 Summarize high reliability organizing as a framework for high reliability safety leadership (*understanding*).

5.3 Explain leadership strategies to build a high reliability "fearless workplace" (*applying*).

Preparation

Prior to completion of the learning activity, you should:

- Read Chapter 5.
- Read *The Fearless Organization: Creating Psychological Safety in the Workplace for Learning, Innovation, and Growth*, by Amy Edmondson.
- Consider various safety leadership styles and their influence on safety leadership actions.
- Consider the role of psychological safety in an HRO.

Instructions

5.1 Interview a local leader at your facility using the following questions and record your answers in Table 5.1. Be prepared to share with your colleagues.

TABLE 5.1 SAFETY LEADERSHIP INTERVIEW QUESTIONS

Interview Questions	Response Notes
What events in your life have had the most positive impact on your leadership and strategic thinking development? What has had the most negative impact?	
What other events, programs, or education have had the most impact on your leadership and patient safety thinking?	
What is your most important core belief that guides the way you lead?	

continues

TABLE 5.1 SAFETY LEADERSHIP INTERVIEW QUESTIONS (CONT.)

Interview Questions	Response Notes
How do you factor in culture, diversity, or other differences into your leadership?	
How do you adapt your leadership to accommodate different age groups?	
What strategies have you used to develop a deeper sense of ownership in your followers' work and in their organization?	
How do you inspire others to achieve more than they expected?	
When you have had a significant setback at work, how did you respond? What did you learn from that setback?	
What are some of the methods you have used to foster safety thinking among peers, followers, and other leaders?	
When you look for the best candidate for a leadership role, what do you consider the most important characteristics?	

5.2 Describe the influence of the local leader's leadership style along with safety leadership actions on organizational quality and safety. Use Table 5.2 to record your answers.

TABLE 5.2 SAFETY LEADERSHIP STYLE INFLUENCE AND ACTION

Leadership Style	Supporting Notes From Interview
Description	

CHAPTER 5 SAFETY LEADERSHIP: COMMITMENT TO HIGH RELIABILITY ORGANIZING

Leadership Style	Supporting Notes From Interview
Attributes	
Behaviors	
Safety leadership actions	

5.3 Go to the following link and complete the leadership assessment: https://www.mindtools.com/pages/article/leadership-style-quiz.htm.

Based on your leadership style, discuss how you would use high reliability organizing as a framework for your high reliability safety leadership style, using Table 5.3 to record your responses. Include specific strategies for each of the five high reliability principles that may assist you as a leader to move in the direction toward high reliability.

TABLE 5.3 MY HIGH RELIABILITY SAFETY LEADERSHIP STYLE AND STRATEGIES

Leadership Style Description:	
High Reliability Organizing Framework	*Leadership Strategies*
Leadership preoccupation with failure	
Leadership reluctance to simplify	

continues

TABLE 5.3 MY HIGH RELIABILITY SAFETY LEADERSHIP STYLE AND STRATEGIES (CONT.)

Leadership Style Description:	
Leadership sensitivity to operations	
Leadership commitment to resilience	
Leadership deference to expertise	

5.4 As a high reliability organizing leader, apply Edmondson's three-phase leadership strategy to build a fearless organization. Include psychological safety, healthy work environment, and fearless workplace in your discussion. Use Table 5.4 to record your responses.

TABLE 5.4 THREE-PHASE LEADERSHIP STRATEGY

Leadership Strategy Phase	Leadership Strategies
Phase I: Setting the Stage	
Phase II: Inviting Participation	
Phase III: Responding Appropriately	

CHAPTER 6

HEALTH EQUITY AND HIGH RELIABILITY: CONNECTING THE DOTS FOR PATIENT SAFETY

In this chapter, you will learn about the relationship between health equity and high reliability. You will also learn how to incorporate health equity concepts into patient safety and quality work.

Learning Objective

Explain how combining health equity and high reliability principles make patient safety and quality work meaningful for patient populations.

Learning Activity 6.1: Use Health Equity Knowledge to Inform Patient Safety Initiatives

Learning Activity Objectives

6.1 Relate ethical frameworks to provide equitable care (*understanding*).

6.2 Articulate ways to address challenges in promoting equitable care (*applying*).

6.3 Defend the importance of addressing root causes of health disparities as a way to promote patient safety (*evaluating*).

6.4 Compile the links between health equity and HRO principles (*creating*).

Preparation

Prior to completion of the learning activity, you should:

- Read Chapter 6
- Read "From HRO to HERO: Making Health Equity a Core System Capability" at https://doi.org/10.1097/JMQ.0000000000000020

Instructions

6.1 Select one of the following ethical frameworks or approaches for decision-making and write one or two paragraphs explaining why the selected framework compels actions that promote health equity. Resource: https://www.pbs.org/wnet/religionandethics/files/2008/09/five_sources.pdf

- Utilitarianism
- Rights-based ethics
- Fairness and justice approach
- The common good approach
- Virtue ethics

_____
_____
_____
_____
_____
_____

6.2 Create a one-page SBAR to explain the concern, give some background, and provide an assessment and recommendations for the following situation.

You received a complaint from a Latinx patient who states the hospital staff was disrespectful and provided biased care because he is an immigrant. He was not offered interpretation and was made to wait in the ED waiting room longer than other people who came in after him. The patient believes he received poor treatment because in the current political climate immigrants are not welcomed. You want to communicate this to your supervisor and make recommendations that will support both staff and community members.

6.3 You have been asked to do an interview where you will defend the following premise: Addressing the root causes of health disparities is important for sustaining health equity work and for patient safety.

Record yourself answering the following interview questions:

- What are the root causes of health disparities?
- Can you speak to one specific patient, provider, system, or social factor that is at the root of health disparities and tell us why it is important to address it and share best practices for addressing it?
- Why is addressing the root causes of health disparities, like discrimination, essential to patient safety?

6.4 Reflect on the links between health equity and high reliability principles to complete the following statements:

- When looking at health equity, *preoccupation with failure* means:

  _____
  _____
  _____

- I can demonstrate *reluctance to simply* when addressing health disparities by:

  _____
  _____
  _____

- One way to practice the principle of *sensitivity to operations* when looking at existing disparities within a system is:

  _____
  _____
  _____

- HROs can demonstrate *deference to expertise* by:

  _____
  _____
  _____

- *Commitment to resilience* related to health equity is evident in an organization when:

  _____
  _____
  _____

PART II

HRO CONCEPTS AND APPLICATION TO PRACTICE: PREOCCUPATION WITH FAILURE

Learning Objective

Recommend quality and safety activities based on high reliability principles (*evaluating*).

Contents

Chapter 7   Using Failure Mode and Effects Analysis to Predict Failure 25

Chapter 8   Paying Attention to Close Calls and Near Misses 29

CHAPTER 7

USING FAILURE MODE AND EFFECTS ANALYSIS TO PREDICT FAILURE

In this chapter, you will learn about anticipation of failure in an HRO. You will also learn about the purpose, potential uses, and challenges of completing a Failure Mode and Effects Analysis (FMEA).

Learning Objective

Explain and discuss the vital role of anticipation of failure in an HRO.

Learning Activity 7.1: Discuss the Importance of the FMEA Process Within a High Reliability Organization

Learning Activity Objectives

7.1 Describe the use of the FMEA as a cornerstone of high reliability (*understanding*).

7.2 Discuss various applications of the FMEA in healthcare (*understanding*).

7.3 Apply concepts of the FMEA to explore potential failures within practice (*applying*).

Preparation

Prior to completion of the learning activity, you should:

- Read Chapter 7.
- Search the literature and find and read one article that uses FMEA as an improvement method.
- Review "Guidance for Performing Failure Mode and Effects Analysis With Performance Improvement Projects" at https://www.cms.gov/Medicare/Provider-Enrollment-and-Certification/QAPI/Downloads/GuidanceForFMEA.pdf.
- Read "Systems Thinking, Culture of Reliability and Safety" at https://www.icesi.edu.co/blogs/pslunes122/files/2012/08/Systems-thinking-culture-of-reliability-and-safety1.pdf.
- Think about the concept of safety imagination and how safety imagination is a key process for high reliability.

Instructions

7.1 List at least four possible opportunities to use FMEA within your practice setting.

1. _____

2. _____

3. _____

4. _____

Discuss why you believe the process is right for an FMEA, including the high-risk nature of the process and the potential for failures. Who would you involve?

_____

_____

_____

_____

_____

_____

7.2 Within your facility, find applications of the FMEA process and list the process examined, failures found, and solutions suggested, using Table 7.1 to record your answers. If your facility has not completed an FMEA, use an article found in the literature as your source.

TABLE 7.1 APPLYING THE FMEA PROCESS

Process Examined	Main Failure Modes	Solutions Suggested	Positive Impact of the FMEA on the Process

7.3 Practice brainstorming failure modes: Select a common process and select one step in the process. List all the ways that the step could fail, the effect of the failure, and the reason for the failure, using Table 7.2 to record your answers.

TABLE 7.2 FAILURE MODES EXAMPLE

How Could This Step Fail?	What Would Happen to the Patient or System if the Step Failed?	Why Would This Step Fail? (Describe the human or system reason.)

7.4 Discuss the importance of psychological safety when brainstorming failure modes within a group.

_____

_____

_____

_____

_____

CHAPTER 8

PAYING ATTENTION TO CLOSE CALLS AND NEAR MISSES

In this chapter, you will learn about why reporting close calls, near misses, and unsafe conditions is the best opportunity to anticipate and fix failures before harm is caused to a patient or system.

Learning Objective

Discuss how the identification and mitigation of near misses, close calls, and unsafe conditions promotes high reliability.

Learning Activity 8.1: Evaluate the Importance of Near Misses, Close Calls, and Unsafe Conditions to High Reliability

Learning Activity Objectives

8.1 Define near miss, close call, and unsafe condition (*remembering*).

8.2 Describe the importance of identifying near misses and close calls to improve safety (*understanding*).

8.3 Discuss barriers to reporting and acting on near misses and close calls within the current environment (*understanding*).

Preparation

- Read Chapter 8.
- Read "Nurses' Experiences in Voluntary Error Reporting: An Integrative Literature Review" at https://doi.org/10.1016/j.ijnss.2021.07.004.
- Read "Reporting and Responding to Patient Safety Incidents Based on Data From Hospitals' Reporting Systems: A Systematic Review" at https://doi.org/10.5430/jha.v9n2p22.

Instructions

8.1 Ask three coworkers to identify a recent near miss, close call, or unsafe condition that they think might lead to patient harm in the near future.

- Ask if they have reported the issue through a formal reporting system. Why or why not?
- What was done to remedy the situation?
- Ask if they are currently aware of "workarounds" to get things done.
- Do they consider the "workaround" an issue worth reporting?

Notes:

_____

_____

_____

_____

8.2 Discuss barriers and facilitators to reporting near misses, close calls, or unsafe conditions.

_____

_____

_____

_____

8.3 Discuss three strategies to make reporting events easier and more useful to improve patient safety.

1. _____

_____

2. _____

_____

3. _____

_____

PART III

HRO CONCEPTS AND APPLICATION TO PRACTICE: RELUCTANCE TO SIMPLIFY

Learning Objective

Recommend quality and safety activities based on high reliability principles (*evaluating*).

Contents

Chapter 9   Human Factors Engineering for Reducing and Recovering From Error 33

Chapter 10 Root Cause Analysis: A Tool for High Reliability in a Complex Environment..36

Chapter 11 Fostering Just Culture in High Reliability Organizations: How Far Have We Come? 39

CHAPTER

9

HUMAN FACTORS ENGINEERING FOR REDUCING AND RECOVERING FROM ERROR

In this chapter, you will learn about the scope and practice of human factors engineering (HFE). You will also learn about the value of partnering with trained HFE practitioners in their efforts to improve patient safety as well as the safety of those on the front lines of healthcare.

Learning Objective

Explore the value of HFE to improve the safety of patients and clinicians.

Learning Activity 9.1: Explain Human Factors Engineering (HFE): The Science and Practice of Designing Work Systems to Fit the Needs, Limitations, and Capabilities of Humans

Learning Activity Objectives

9.1 Discuss how practitioners of HFE think about work systems (*understanding*).

9.2 Explain how the design of the work system can make it easier for errors to occur and harder to recover from (*applying*).

9.3 Explain how practitioners of HFE approach redesigning the work system to reduce opportunities for error and to facilitate recovery from error (*analyzing*).

Preparation

Prior to completion of the learning activity, you should:

- Read Chapter 9.
- Read "SEIPS 2.0: A Human Factors Framework for Studying and Improving the Work of Healthcare Professionals and Patients" at https://doi.org/10.1080/00140139.2013.83864.
- Read "Process Mapping—The Foundation for Effective Quality Improvement" at https://doi.org/10.1016/j.cppeds.2018.08.010.

Instructions

9.1 Identify an error-prone process for improvement at your organization.

9.2 Form a group to map out the current process targeted for improvement.

9.3 Identify characteristics of work system elements (persons, tools/technology, tasks, physical environment, and organizational environment) that make it easier/harder for errors to happen, using Table 9.1 to record your group's answers. Include learning from error in your discussion.

TABLE 9.1 ERROR-PRONE PROCESS FOR IMPROVEMENT

Work System Element Characteristics (persons, tools/technology, tasks, physical environment, organizational environment)	Easier for Errors to Happen? Why?	Harder for Errors to Happen? Why?	Learning From Error

9.4 Brainstorm corrective actions that target/leverage these characteristics and do not rely heavily on things like training, instructions for use, and warnings to work, using Table 9.2.

TABLE 9.2 CORRECTIVE ACTIONS BRAINSTORMING

Work Element Characteristic	Corrective Action

9.5 Discuss the types of human errors that most commonly occur. Give examples and a possible solution from a human factor's perspective using Table 9.3 to record your answers.

TABLE 9.3 TYPES OF HUMAN FACTOR ERRORS

Type of Human Factor Error	Definition	Example	HFE Solution
Skill-based error			
Rule-based error			
Knowledge-based error			

CHAPTER 10

ROOT CAUSE ANALYSIS: A TOOL FOR HIGH RELIABILITY IN A COMPLEX ENVIRONMENT

In this chapter, you will learn about the background, processes, and challenges of using root cause analysis (RCA) as a tool to advance safety in an HRO. You will also learn the steps in an effective RCA.

Learning Objective

Explore the usefulness and challenges of using RCA as a tool to advance safety in an HRO.

Learning Activity 10.1: Discuss Use of RCA as a Tool for Embedding the High Reliability Principle "Reluctance to Simplify" Into a Safety Event Investigation

Learning Activity Objectives

10.1 Discuss the significance of using RCA as a tool to discover system issues (*understanding*).

10.2 Apply the "Five Whys" questioning technique to a familiar problem (*applying*).

10.3 Discuss common problems that may lessen RCA effectiveness (*understanding*).

10.4 Explain how bias occurs and how to avoid bias during the RCA process (*understanding*).

Preparation

Prior to completion of the learning activity, you should:

- Read Chapter 10.
- Read "RCA_2 Improving Root Cause Analysis and Actions to Prevent Harm" at https://www.med.unc.edu/ihqi/files/2018/07/RCA2-National-Patient-Safety-Foundation.pdf.

Instructions

10.1 Read the case examples regarding the errors in the first few pages of the chapter. Identify the active errors and latent errors in the mistake, using Table 10.1 to record your answers.

TABLE 10.1 ACTIVE AND LATENT ERRORS

	Active Error (human error)	Latent Error (system issues)
Medication error: Antibiotic given too quickly		
Ordering error: Two patients received incorrect radiology tests		
Medication error: Gave insulin instead of antibiotic		

10.2 Discuss the impact to high reliability when system issues are identified and corrected rather than correcting the individual only. Reflect on a time in your career when an individual was blamed/disciplined for an event. How did that affect the overall culture of safety? Did the error recur?

_____

_____

_____

_____

_____

_____

10.3 Identify a safety issue: Practice asking "Five Whys" to get to the root cause. The first "why" addresses the one most proximate to the error, usually a clinician. The last "why" question should be at the system level (use Figure 10.1 to record your answers).

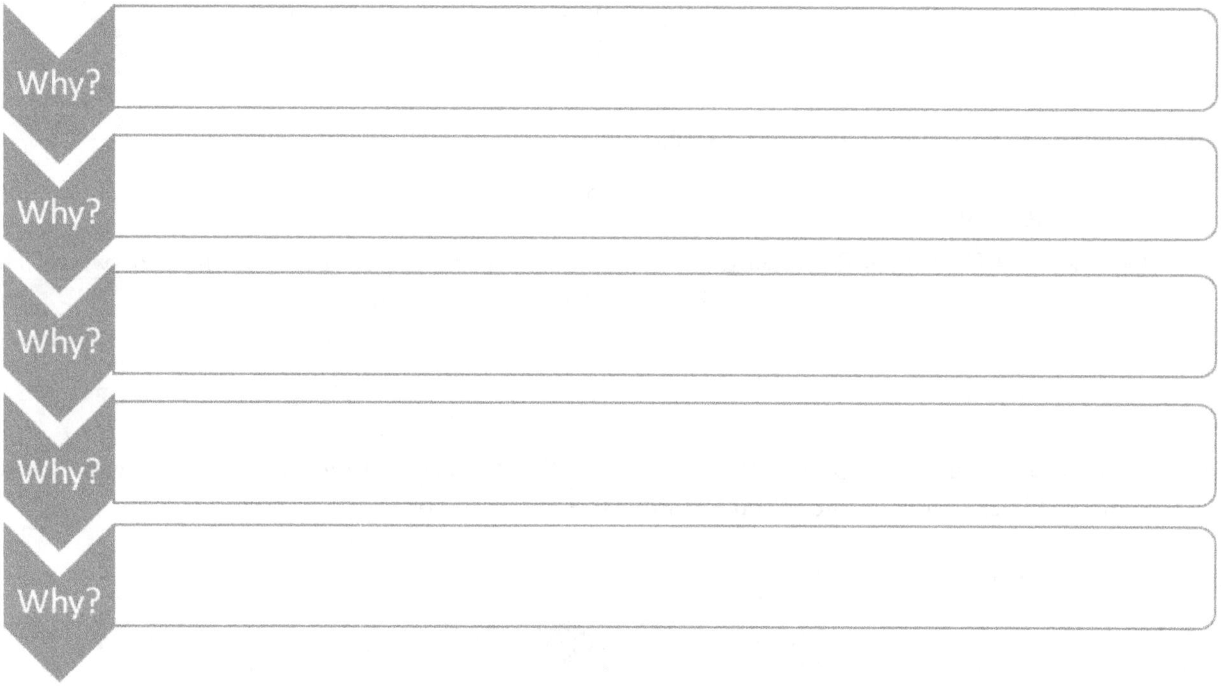

Why? _____

Why? _____

Why? _____

Why? _____

Why? _____

FIGURE 10.1 Practicing the "Five Whys" to identify causes of error.

10.4 List three strategies to ensure RCA is effective to identify root cause.

1. _____

_____

2. _____

_____

3. _____

_____

CHAPTER 11

FOSTERING JUST CULTURE IN HIGH RELIABILITY ORGANIZATIONS: HOW FAR HAVE WE COME?

In this chapter, you will learn about Just Culture. You will also learn about the challenges of Just Culture in practice due to outcome bias, misapplication of assumptions, and application of the Just Culture algorithm without a clear commitment to the tenets of the culture change needed to learn from errors.

Learning Objective

Discover the history, theory, and challenges of implementing Just Culture in practice.

Learning Activity 11.1: Examine the Features and Challenges of a Just Culture Within a Highly Reliable Safety Program and the Current Healthcare Environment

Learning Activity Objectives

11.1 Compare and contrast a Just Culture versus a blameless culture versus a punitive culture (*analyzing*).

11.2 Apply Just Culture principles to examples (*applying*).

11.3 Discuss challenges to a Just Culture (*understanding*).

11.4 Describe the differences between a retributive Just Culture and a restorative Just Culture (*understanding*).

11.5 Discuss the challenge of Just Culture when the patient outcome is "bad" (*applying*).

Preparation

Prior to completion of the learning activity, you should:

- Read Chapter 11.
- Watch the video *Annie's Story* at https://youtu.be/zeldVu-3DpM.
- Find and read an article on second victim syndrome. Option: "Second Victims in Health Care: Current Perspectives" at https://doi.org/10.2147/AMEP.S185912.
- Read "Restorative Just Culture Checklist" at https://safetydifferently.com/restorative-just-culture-checklist/restorativejustculturechecklist-2/.
- Read "Reckless Homicide at Vanderbilt? A Just Culture Analysis" at https://www.linkedin.com/pulse/reckless-homicide-vanderbilt-just-culture-analysis-david-marx/.

Instructions

11.1 Discuss the differences between a blameless culture, a punitive culture, and a Just Culture and the effects to patient safety for each type of culture.

_____

_____

_____

_____

_____

_____

11.2 Define the three types of errors that can occur and give examples from your experience using Table 11.1 to record your answers.

TABLE 11.1 EXAMPLE OF DEFINING THE THREE TYPES OF ERRORS

	Definition	Example in Practice	How Is This Normally Dealt With?	How Could It Be Dealt With to Promote a Just Culture?
Human error				
Risky behavior				
Reckless behavior				

11.3 Interview a manager within your organization. Find out the following:
- Current Just Culture algorithm used in the facility
- How the manager was trained to use the algorithm
- Example of how the algorithm has been used to promote positive learning
- Whether there is a second victim program or a support system for those involved in errors
- Any difficulties in applying the Just Culture process, especially when the outcome of the error was serious

11.4 Discuss the impact of involvement in an error to the healthcare provider.

_____

_____

_____

Describe second victim syndrome and the effect to the individual and the healthcare system.

_____

_____

_____

Discuss how a restorative Just Culture can assist in healing the individual involved in the error and can affect system safety and healing.

_____

_____

_____

11.5 Discuss challenges to Just Culture and outcome bias when the outcome is catastrophic. Reflect on the Vanderbilt case or another case involving litigation or media coverage. How does the outcome bias affect the application of Just Culture?

_____

_____

_____

_____

_____

_____

PART IV

HRO CONCEPTS AND APPLICATION TO PRACTICE: SENSITIVITY TO OPERATIONS

Learning Objective

Recommend quality and safety activities based on high reliability principles (*evaluating*).

Contents

Chapter 12   Alarm Safety: Working Solutions...44

Chapter 13   Innovative Technology, Standardization, and the Impact
on High Reliability..47

Chapter 14   Tiered Safety Huddles...51

CHAPTER 12

ALARM SAFETY: WORKING SOLUTIONS

In this chapter, you will learn about improvements directed toward alarm safety in response to harm related to alarm fatigue, increased technology, and regulatory guidance. You will also learn about interventions based on high reliability principles as a strategy for sustainable alarm safety.

Learning Objective

Explore the high-risk nature of clinical alarm management and the challenges of identifying and containing the risk to prevent adverse events.

Learning Activity 12.1: Appraise the Concept of Alarm Fatigue and the Possibilities for Improvement When Applying High Reliability Principles to Clinical Alarm Safety

Learning Activity Objectives

12.1 Consider the implications of alarm fatigue within the clinical environment (*understanding*).

12.2 Apply concepts of failure mode effects analysis (FMEA) to appraise clinical alarms within a practice environment (*applying*).

Preparation

Prior to completion of the learning activity, you should:

- Read Chapter 12.
- Read "A Call to Alarms: Current State and Future Directions in the Battle Against Alarm Fatigue" at https://www.ncbi.nlm.nih.gov/pmc/articles/PMC6263784/pdf/nihms-1502834.pdf.

Instructions

12.1 In a 500-word essay, define alarm fatigue, give examples, and discuss the implications for patient safety and high reliability.

- Include examples of actionable versus nonactionable alarms and the implication for alarm fatigue.
- Describe how healthcare organizations are improving the safety of clinical alarms.
- Discuss how these organizations used data to track progress.
- Finally, discuss how high reliability principles and improvement concepts were used in the improvement efforts.
    - Include preoccupation with failure, attention to detail, and deference to expertise.
    - Include standardization and situational awareness.

12.2 Perform an assessment of clinical alarms or noise distraction in your area of experience within an FMEA format, using Table 12.1 to record your answers.

TABLE 12.1 FMEA ANALYSIS OF A CLINICAL ALARM OR NOISE DISTRACTION

Alarm	Expected Response	How Could Response Fail?	What Would Happen to a Patient Due to a Failure?	Why Would This Response Fail?

CHAPTER 13

INNOVATIVE TECHNOLOGY, STANDARDIZATION, AND THE IMPACT ON HIGH RELIABILITY

In this chapter, you will learn how new and innovative technology, automation, standardization, and forcing functions are effective approaches to making a process highly reliable. You will also learn that successful integration of technologies requires a systematic approach, an understanding of the learning health system, and a commitment to patient safety as a foundational value to achieve highly reliable performance.

Learning Objective

Examine how technology can be used to effectively hardwire processes and improve results.

Learning Activity 13.1: Apply Knowledge of Effective Interventions for High Reliability to Analyze Technological Advances in Your Practice

Learning Activity Objectives:

13.1 Discuss technology and its impact on high reliability in your environment (*understanding*).

13.2 Analyze current safety interventions from your experience and place them in the Institute for Safe Medication Practices (ISMP) hierarchy of interventions (*analyzing*).

13.3 Discuss the significance of workarounds, including why workarounds occur and how to mitigate them (*understanding*).

Preparation

Prior to completion of the learning activity, you should:

- Read Chapter 13.
- Read "Nurse Workarounds in the Electronic Health Record: An Integrative Review" at https://doi.org/10.1093/jamia/ocaa050.
- Read "Human Factors Engineering" at https://psnet.ahrq.gov/primer/human-factors-engineering.
- Read "Education as a Low-Value Improvement Intervention: Often Necessary but Rarely Sufficient" at https://doi.org/10.1136/bmjqs-2019-010411.

Instructions

13.1 Assess your work environment. List examples of how technology is used and what impact it has on patient safety and high reliability. Consider the following in the discussion:

- How does the technology improve workflow?
- How does the technology improve communication?
- How does the technology improve patient safety?
- Do end users see the value of the technology?
- Are there any unexpected consequences that were found after implementation?

_____

_____

_____

_____

_____

_____

13.2 Use the ISMP hierarchy and list examples of each level of the hierarchy in relation to your practice and prevention of high-risk events in Table 13.1. Also, list the pros and cons and safety effectiveness of each level.

TABLE 13.1 APPLYING THE ISMP HIERARCHY FOR PREVENTION OF HIGH-RISK EVENTS

	Example in Practice	Pros	Cons	How Does This Improve Individual Safety?	How Does This Improve System Safety?	Will This Prevent the Error From Recurring?
Education and information						
Rules and policies						
Checklists and double-check systems						
Standardization and protocols						
Automation and computerization						
Forcing functions and constraints						

13.3 The goal of high reliability strategies is to make it easier to do the right thing and harder to do the wrong thing. Workarounds are commonly created because it is difficult to do the right thing. Using Table 13.2, discuss workarounds to various practices, why they were created, and how to mitigate them.

TABLE 13.2 ANALYSIS OF WORKAROUNDS

Safety Technology	Workaround	Why Does It Exist?	How Can It Be Fixed?

CHAPTER 14

TIERED SAFETY HUDDLES

In this chapter, you will learn about the concept of a tiered safety huddle as a strategy to maintain an awareness of operational conditions in an HRO. You will also learn about how tiered safety huddles used to ensure problems from the front line of care are escalated to higher levels within the organization for awareness, system accountability, and resolution of the problem.

Learning Objective

Examine the tiered safety huddle as a vehicle to increase organization and system situational awareness.

Learning Activity 14.1: Describe the Value of the Tiered Huddle in Healthcare as an Effective Tool to Promote High Reliability in a Complex Organization

Learning Activity Objectives

14.1 Describe the purpose and the value of a tiered huddle to patient safety and quality (*understanding*).

14.2 Appraise the tiered huddle intervention as an effective tool within a complex environment (*analyzing*).

Preparation

Prior to completion of the learning activity, you should:

- Read Chapter 14.
- Read "Tiered Safety Huddles Target Zero Harm" at https://www.todayshospitalist.com/tiered-safety-huddles-target-zero-harm/.
- Read "Creating a Process for the Implementation of Tiered Huddles in a Veterans Affairs Medical Center" at https://doi.org/10.1093/milmed/usac073.

Instructions

14.1 Assess your current work environment or interview a clinician in a healthcare work environment using the following questions. Use Table 14.1 to record your answers.

TABLE 14.1 PROBLEM AND ERROR IDENTIFICATION FOR FRONTLINE CARE PROVIDERS

Interview Questions	Response Notes
How are problems surfaced by those at the front line of care?	
How often do those from the front line bring up issues?	
Is there a formal mechanism to ensure these issues are recorded and escalated to those who can resolve the problems?	
Are your senior leaders aware of the daily challenges at the front line of care?	
Are senior leaders made aware of these challenges on a daily basis?	

Interview Questions	Response Notes
What is the senior leader's role and response to resolve daily challenges?	
How does the resolution make it back to the front line?	
How do issues that involve the "system"—such as complex processes and procedures, equipment issues, and contract issues—get resolved?	
How are problems surfaced by those at the front line of care?	
How often do those from the front line bring up issues?	

14.2 Search the literature to consider healthcare as a complex system. Discuss the following:

- Define a complex system.
- List characteristics of healthcare systems that contribute to complexity.
- Discuss how a tiered huddle contributes to all principles of high reliability.
- How does a tiered huddle provide a mechanism to handle aspects of complexity?

_____
_____
_____
_____
_____
_____
_____

PART V

HRO CONCEPTS AND APPLICATION TO PRACTICE: DEFERENCE TO EXPERTISE

Learning Objective

Recommend quality and safety activities based on high reliability principles (*evaluating*).

Contents

Chapter 15 The Current Need for Interprofessional Collaborative Care and Teamwork 55

Chapter 16 Meaningful Patient Engagement: Best Practice for High Reliability 58

Chapter 17 Pediatric Patient Safety: Utilizing Safety Coaching as a Strategy Toward Zero Harm 61

CHAPTER 15

THE CURRENT NEED FOR INTERPROFESSIONAL COLLABORATIVE CARE AND TEAMWORK

In this chapter, you will learn about how an increased focus on quality, safety, and efficiency in healthcare has placed greater attention on understanding the complexity of healthcare teams. You will also learn about interprofessional collaboration and teamwork in the context of HROs.

Learning Objective

Illustrate interprofessional collaboration and teamwork in the context of HROs.

Learning Activity 15.1: Describe and Explain an Interprofessional Team in the Context of HROs

Learning Activity Objectives

15.1 Describe interprofessional collaboration in the context of HROs (*understanding*).

15.2 Explain teamwork in the context of HROs (*applying*).

Preparation

Prior to completion of the learning activity, you should:

- Read Chapter 15.
- Read "Teamwork in Healthcare: Key Discoveries Enabling Safer, High-Quality Care" at https://doi.org/10.1037/amp0000298.
- Read "Creating a Culture of Teamwork Through the Use of the TeamSTEPPS Framework: A Review of the Literature and Considerations for Nurse Practitioners" at https://doi.org/10.12806/V21/I1/R11.
- Consider characteristics of effective interprofessional teams.
- Consider evidence-based tools that support teams in assessing the current state to best identify short-term goals for improving team function.

Instructions

15.1 Describe the characteristics of an interprofessional collaborative team in your organization. Include an assessment of the strength and weaknesses of the team using one evidence-based tool. Use Table 15.1 to record your responses.

TABLE 15.1 INTERPROFESSIONAL COLLABORATIVE TEAM ASSESSMENT

Interprofessional Team Name:

Team Characteristics	Description

Team Assessment Using the Evidence-Based Assessment Tool:	
Strengths	**Weaknesses**

15.2 Based on your assessment, make recommendations on how to strengthen the performance of the interprofessional collaborative team in the context of an HRO. Include one team training strategy and rationale for use. Use Table 15.2 to record your responses.

TABLE 15.2 RECOMMENDATIONS FOR INTERPROFESSIONAL COLLABORATIVE TEAM IMPROVEMENT

Weakness	Recommendation for Improvement (include team training strategy with rationale)	High Reliability Context (link to high reliability principles)

CHAPTER 16

MEANINGFUL PATIENT ENGAGEMENT: BEST PRACTICE FOR HIGH RELIABILITY

In this chapter, you will learn about healthcare organizations' focus on meaningful patient engagement in the context of high reliability efforts such as quality and safety improvement. You will also learn about methods commonly used to partner with patients and families, as well as practical strategies to approximate and sustain partnerships.

Learning Objective

Explore how partnership and collaboration with patients contributes to the achievement of a consistent, highly reliable patient experience.

Learning Activity 16.1: Explain Meaningful Patient and Family Engagement In The Context Of High Reliability For Patient Safety And Quality

Learning Activity Objectives

16.1 Identify co-producing opportunities for patient and family engagement in an organization (*applying*).

16.2 Analyze various patient and family engagement methodological approaches to create meaningful partnerships in safety and quality improvement (*analyzing*).

Preparation

Prior to completion of the learning activity, you should:

- Read Chapter 16.
- Read "Guide to Patient and Family Engagement in Hospital Quality and Safety" at https://www.ahrq.gov/patient-safety/patients-families/engagingfamilies/index.html.

Instructions

16.1 Describe how to empower patients and families across patient and family engagement opportunities, using Table 16.1 to record your responses.

TABLE 16.1 EXAMPLE: ENGAGING AND EMPOWERING PATIENTS AND FAMILIES

Level of Engagement	Ways to Engage and Empower Patients and Families	Example(s)	Facilitator(s)	Barrier(s)

16.2 In a 500-word essay, discuss how to create meaningful patient and family partnerships in a safety or quality initiative. Identify a safety or quality improvement opportunity from the literature or at your organization and discuss how you could codesign the project to create meaningful patient and family partnerships. Include the following in your discussion:

- Collaborate with senior leaders
- Build trusting relationships and instill confidence
- Recruit and retain participants
- Empower the voice of patients and families
- Power dynamics
- Diverse perspectives
- Facilitators and barriers

CHAPTER 17

PEDIATRIC PATIENT SAFETY: UTILIZING SAFETY COACHING AS A STRATEGY TOWARD ZERO HARM

In this chapter, you will learn about the difficulty of sustaining successful culture change. You will also learn that taking culture change to the front line through peer safety coaches is an effective intervention to reinforce and sustain zero harm culture.

Learning Objective

Describe implementation of a safety coach program that improved and created a platform for sustainability of HRO principles within a pediatric environment.

Learning Activity 17.1: Examine the Role of Safety Coaches as a Vehicle for Successful Change Management and Sustainability of HRO Principles

Learning Activity Objectives:

17.1 Describe factors that influence change (*remembering*).

17.2 Describe the role of the patient safety coach and why it is needed for high reliability and sustained culture change (*remembering*).

17.3 Examine challenges with peer coaching and suggest solutions (*applying*).

Preparation

Prior to completion of the learning activity, you should:

- Read Chapter 17.
- Read "How Peer Coaching Can Make Work Less Lonely" at https://hbr.org/2018/10/how-peer-coaching-can-make-work-less-lonely.
- Watch the video *Peer to Peer Coaching* at https://www.ahrq.gov/hai/cusp/videos/07d-peer-2-peer-coach/index.html.
- Read "Leading Change: Why Transformation Efforts Fail" at https://hbr.org/1995/03/leading-change-why-transformation-efforts-fail-2.

Instructions

17.1 Describe a recent initiative that succeeded or failed within your organization. Correlate the success or failure to characteristics within a change model.
- What was the initiative?
- Who led the initiative?
- How was the initiative received at the front line?
- What tactics were used to spread the initiative and sustain the progress? Was a change model used? Which one?
- Did the tactics succeed? Why?

- Review the Kotter article. What failure factors from the article were evident in a failure or mitigated in a success? What could have been done differently?

_____

_____

_____

_____

_____

_____

17.2 Examine the role of the safety coach and how safety coaches can create sustainability of a zero-harm initiative.

- Find and discuss a definition of a healthcare patient safety coach.
- What are the challenges with giving feedback to peers?
- Which is more successful: positive or negative feedback?
- What kind of training do safety coaches need?
- How can the role be supported to sustain gains in patient safety and quality?
- Describe the benefits to a safety coach program within an organization to achieve a culture change to high reliability. How is coaching from a peer different from coaching from a supervisor?

_____

_____

_____

_____

_____

_____

17.3 Practice safety coaching using an example from Table 17.1 or your own example to reinforce a desired safety behavior.

TABLE 17.1 PRACTICING SAFETY COACHING

	What Did You Observe?	What Is the Expectation?	How Would You Coach?
Hand hygiene: Staff member does not practice hand hygiene.			
Preventions of falls: Staff member leaves the room and does not set the bed alarm.			
Protecting confidentiality: You hear staff members talking about a patient in the elevator.			
Effective communication: You witness a peer using a repeat-back to clarify an order.			
Asking questions: You hear a peer clarifying an unclear order.			

PART VI

HRO CONCEPTS AND APPLICATION TO PRACTICE: COMMITMENT TO RESILIENCE

Learning Objective

Recommend quality and safety activities based on high reliability principles (*evaluating*).

Contents

Chapter 18 Designing Resilience Into the Work Environment 66

Chapter 19 Building High Reliability Through Simulation 69

Chapter 20 Building Resilience Through Team Training: Rapid Response and In-Hospital Cardiac Arrests Events 71

Chapter 21 Sustaining a Culture of Safety 75

CHAPTER 18

DESIGNING RESILIENCE INTO THE WORK ENVIRONMENT

In this chapter, you will learn about a social-ecological perspective of resilience. You will also learn to relate this perspective to high reliability, design a resilient work environment, and associate individual and work environment resilience with clinician well-being.

Learning Objective

Discover a social-ecological perspective of resilience to support clinician well-being.

Learning Activity 18.1: Apply a Social-Ecological Perspective of Resilience to Support Clinician Well-Being in the Work Environment

Learning Activity Objectives

18.1 Describe resilience and how it relates to high reliability (*understanding*).

18.2 Discuss opportunities for designing a resilient work environment (*understanding*).

18.3 Associate individual and work environment resilience with clinician well-being (*understanding*).

Preparation

Prior to completion of the learning activity, you should:

- Read Chapter 18.

- Read *Taking Action Against Clinician Burnout: A Systems Approach to Professional Well-Being* at https://doi.org/10.17226/25521.

Instructions

18.1 Describe resilience in your organization in the context of high reliability.

_____

_____

_____

18.2 Discuss three strategies to design a more resilient work environment in your organization. Include tactics to facilitate clinician well-being, using Table 18.1 to record your answers.

TABLE 18.1 EXAMPLE OF STRATEGIES TO DESIGN A RESILIENT WORK ENVIRONMENT

Work Environment Resilience Strategy	Tactics to Facilitate Clinician Well-Being
1.	
2.	
3.	

18.3 In Table 18.2, give three examples of how individual and work environment resilience affect clinician well-being within a social-ecological perspective of resilience.

TABLE 18.2 EFFECTS OF INDIVIDUAL AND WORK ENVIRONMENT RESILIENCE

Social-Ecological Perspective	Individual Resilience	Workplace Environment Resilience	Clinician Well-Being Influence
Individual			
Team resilience			
Organization resilience			
Society/external environment			

CHAPTER 19

BUILDING HIGH RELIABILITY THROUGH SIMULATION

In this chapter, you will learn about healthcare simulation and blend simulation with the concepts of high reliability to create a view of simulation that improves the safety of high-risk processes. You will also learn about the benefits of employing simulation as an advanced quality improvement and patient safety tool.

Learning Objective

Describe the emergence of simulation in hospitals, schools, and other healthcare organizations as an advanced quality-improvement and patient-safety tool.

Learning Activity 19.1: Explore Opportunities to Use Simulation to Improve Safety and Reliability of Risk-Prone Processes

Learning Activity Objectives

19.1 Compare and contrast traditional simulation and simulation designed for high reliability (*analyzing*).

19.2 Apply simulation to a high-risk process to improve the safety of the process (*applying*).

Preparation

Prior to completion of the learning activity, you should:

- Read Chapter 19.
- Read "Using Clinical Simulation to Study How to Improve Quality and Safety in Healthcare" at https://doi.org/10.1136/bmjstel-2018-000370.
- Find one peer-reviewed research article that applies simulation to a clinical safety or quality problem.

Instructions

19.1 In a 500-word essay, describe the difference between traditional simulation, such as experience for learning competencies, and simulation to improve safety of a high-risk process.

- List some high-risk processes from your experience that might benefit from a simulation exercise.
- How have these processes been practiced or simulated in your organization?
- Were the practice sessions realistic?
- Did the practice identify areas for improvement in teamwork, communication, or critical thinking?
- Did the practice identify potential failures that might occur in the process?
- Did participants in the practice session feel psychologically safe to speak up?
- Did debriefing occur after the practice session?
- Pick one of the high-risk processes that you currently practice or drill in your facility. Redesign the practice or drill to create a simulation that identifies safety issues within the process and increases the safety of the process.
- Describe how simulation could be combined with an FMEA to identify failure modes.

19.2 Present your research article to fellow students:

- What was the practice problem that the simulation addressed?
- Describe the method used for simulation.
- What were the objectives and outcomes of the simulation?
- Identify a high reliability principle that the simulation addressed or could have addressed.

CHAPTER 20

BUILDING RESILIENCE THROUGH TEAM TRAINING: RAPID RESPONSE AND IN-HOSPITAL CARDIAC ARREST EVENTS

In this chapter, you will assess and evaluate the role resilience plays through team training events. You will practice with an in-depth example of a healthcare emergency where multiple team members manage the emergency.

Learning Objective

Explain and evaluate how the high reliability principle of resilience improves team response to a cardiac event.

Learning Activity 20.1: Evaluate Rapid Response and In-Hospital Cardiac Arrest Event Team Performance

Learning Activity Objectives

20.1 Evaluate rapid response and in-hospital cardiac arrest event team performance (*evaluating*).

20.2 Explain team resilience gap analysis (*analyzing*).

Preparation

Prior to completion of the learning activity, you should:

- Read Chapter 20.
- Read "Empowering Nurses to Activate the Rapid Response Team" at https://doi.org/10.1097/01.NURSE.0000662356.08413.90.

Instructions

20.1 Prepare an in-hospital cardiac arrest event team debrief using the post-code pause structured format (see Figure 20.1). Include team resilience gap analysis in your discussion.

Post-Code Pause Reflection

Date: _____ Age of Patient: _____ Type of Alert: _____

**Names of all staff members involved in post resuscitation pause

**After the Event, everyone pauses for 10 seconds of silence to either remember the life of the person or celebrate the success of the Code Blue

What did the team do well?

What intervention(s) do you wish had or had not been offered?

How is your satisfaction with the equipment and medications available?

Where can we grow and improve?

How did we support the family (if they are present)?

How are you doing after the code?

What do you need to be able to be successful for returning to work right now?

Additional comments or concerns:

FIGURE 20.1 Post-code pause form.

20.2 Prepare a rapid response event team debrief using the "What's Right?" structured format. Include team resilience gap analysis in your discussion (see Table 20.1). The team leader will ask:

- Identify two things that went well in this RRT.
- Identify anything we can do to improve our RRT.

Each team member will be encouraged to share thoughts and new ideas.

TABLE 20.1 RESILIENCE QUALITIES TO CONSIDER DURING GAP ANALYSIS

Indicator	Present	Absent	Follow-Up	Outcome Date
Are red-flag events or near misses reported?				
Is reporting of red-flag events rewarded?				
Is reporting of red-flag events punished?				
Have suggestions for workflow come from the workforce level?				
Do team meetings allow time for open discussion of everyday processes?				
Is the workflow regularly observed and evaluated by others?				
Does this process allow variation, or is variation open to safety issues?				
Have there been action-based mock drills?				
Are preprocess briefings used regularly?				
Are post-event debriefings used regularly?				
Is crew resource management training used with supervisors, and are the results monitored by leadership?				
Are stressful events (with or without outcome errors) reviewed?				
Are predictable workforce stressors identified and mitigated?				
After error mitigation, is the goal to return to steady state?				
Are the values of safety supported on every level of the workforce?				
Is data about safety, productivity, or processes well known and understood at all levels of the workforce?				

CHAPTER 21

SUSTAINING A CULTURE OF SAFETY

In this chapter, you will learn how resilient organizations can sustain a culture of safety by creating an organizational culture of personal and professional accountability.

Learning Objective

Explore a framework for change with strategies to sustain and maintain the gains within a culture of safety.

Learning Activity 21.1: Focus on Sustaining a Culture of Safety in a Resilient Organization

Learning Activity Objectives

21.1 Discuss organizational vulnerabilities, related performance, and adherence to regulations and policies across the care continuum as a rationale for sustaining a culture of safety (*understanding*).

21.2 Apply a framework for change to sustain and maintain a culture of safety (*applying*).

21.3 Explain strategies to maintain the gains within a culture of safety in a resilient organization (*analyzing*).

Preparation

Prior to completion of the learning activity, you should:

- Read Chapter 21.
- Read *It Starts With One: Changing Individuals Changes Organizations*, by J. S. Black.

Instructions

21.1 Discuss steps in developing culture change to support individual professional accountability and healthcare system performance.

_____

_____

_____

_____

21.2 Apply an evidence-based change model of your choice to a problem at your organization. Include barriers to change and mitigation strategies, using Table 21.1 to record your answers.

TABLE 21.1 CHANGE MODEL APPLICATION

Change Model	Barriers to Change	Barrier Mitigation Strategies

Change Model	Barriers to Change	Barrier Mitigation Strategies

21.3 In Table 21.2, name three strategies you could use after an evidence-based change to maintain and sustain gains in a culture of safety.

TABLE 21.2 THREE STRATEGIES FOR GAINS IN A CULTURE OF SAFETY

Strategy	Tactics
1.	
2.	
3.	

PART VII

ASSIMILATION INTO PRACTICE ACROSS THE CONTINUUM

Learning Objective

Integrate high reliability principles into healthcare practice (*creating*).

Contents

Chapter 22 Ambulatory Care: The Frontier for High Reliability 79

Chapter 23 The Synthesis Among Magnet Recognition Program® Model Components and High Reliability Organization Principles 81

Chapter 24 Realizing High Reliability: Nurse Scientist and Bedside Scientist Collaboration 84

Chapter 25 Ensuring High Reliability in Acute Stroke Treatment 87

CHAPTER 22

AMBULATORY CARE: THE FRONTIER FOR HIGH RELIABILITY

In this chapter, you will learn about how high reliability principles can be used to address key quality and safety challenges in ambulatory care. You will learn about the scope of ambulatory services as well as some of the unique complexities and challenges of this specialty.

Learning Objective

Discover how the principles of high reliability can mitigate quality and safety challenges in the ambulatory care setting.

Learning Activity 22.1: Integrate High Reliability Principles to Address Quality and Safety Challenges in Ambulatory Care

Learning Activity Objectives

22.1 Discuss the scope of ambulatory services and the varied ambulatory settings (*understanding*).

22.2 Explain complexities and challenges of ambulatory care (*understanding*).

22.3 Articulate how each of the principles of high reliability can be used to mitigate quality and safety challenges in the ambulatory care space (*applying*).

Preparation

Prior to completion of the learning activity, you should:

- Read Chapter 22.
- Read "The Economics of Patient Safety in Primary and Ambulatory Care: Flying Blind" at https://doi.org/10.1787/baf425ad-en.

Instructions

22.1 Choose an ambulatory care setting in your organization. Include the rationale for your choice. Record your responses in Table 22.1

22.2 Identify at least three complexities and challenges of the chosen ambulatory care setting, adding them to Table 22.1.

22.3 Continuing with Table 22.1, add high reliability principles that can mitigate complexities and challenges of the chosen ambulatory care setting.

TABLE 22.1 APPLYING HIGH RELIABILITY PRINCIPLES IN AMBULATORY CARE SETTINGS

Ambulatory Care Setting:

Rationale:

Complexities	Unique Safety Challenges	High Reliability Solution

CHAPTER 23

THE SYNTHESIS AMONG MAGNET RECOGNITION PROGRAM® MODEL COMPONENTS AND HIGH RELIABILITY ORGANIZATION PRINCIPLES

In this chapter, you will learn about how the Magnet® model component characteristics provide the foundation for synergistic relationships with HRO principles. You will also learn about the synergy of Magnet components and high reliability principles.

Learning Objective

Discover how high reliability principles can be related to the components of the Magnet model.

Learning Activity 23.1: Explain the Synergistic Relationship Between the Magnet Model Components and the Principles of High Reliability

Learning Activity Objectives

23.1 Describe the Magnet Recognition Program components (*understanding*).

23.2 Discuss the synergy of high reliability principles with Magnet Recognition Program components (*understanding*).

Preparation

Prior to completion of the learning activity, you should:

- Read Chapter 23.
- Read "Magnet Model® – Creating a Magnet Culture" at https://www.nursingworld.org/organizational-programs/magnet/magnet-model/.

Instructions

23.1 Discuss the five components and component characteristics of the Magnet model, recording your answers in Table 23.1.

TABLE 23.1 COMPONENTS AND CHARACTERISTICS OF THE MAGNET MODEL

Magnet Component	Description
1.	
2.	
3.	
4.	
5.	

23.2 Describe the synergy of high reliability principles and Magnet Recognition Program components and include examples of synergy, using Table 23.2 to record your responses.

TABLE 23.2 SYNERGY OF HIGH RELIABILITY AND MAGNET RECOGNITION PROGRAM

Magnet Recognition Component/ Description	Example of Magnet Component From Organization	High Reliability Principle	Description of Synergy

CHAPTER 24

REALIZING HIGH RELIABILITY: NURSE SCIENTIST AND BEDSIDE SCIENTIST COLLABORATION

In this chapter, you will learn about the collaborative relationship of bedside scientists and nurse scientists in an HRO. You will also learn about a proposed framework to facilitate organizational quality improvement, evidence-based practice, and research agendas and infrastructure supporting the conduct of nursing research in a highly reliable organization.

Learning Objective

Explain the collaborative, synergistic relationship between nurse scientists and bedside scientists to promote a culture of safety and inquiry in an HRO.

Learning Activity 24.1: Discover the Role of the Nurse Scientist and Bedside Scientist in a High Reliability Organization

Learning Activity Objectives

24.1 Explain the role of the nurse scientist and bedside scientist in an HRO (*understanding*).

24.2 Summarize the collaborative relationship between the nurse scientist and bedside scientist in an HRO (*understanding*).

Preparation

Prior to completion of the learning activity, you should:

- Read Chapter 24.
- Read "How to Improve: Model for Improvement" at https://www.ihi.org/resources/how-improve-model-improvement.
- Read "The Role of the Nurse Scientist and Nursing Research Within a National Integrated Health Care System" at https://doi.org/10.1097/NAQ.0000000000000644.
- Read "Why Nursing Research Matters" at https://doi.org/10.1097/NNA.0000000000001005.
- Read "What Is Evidence-Based Practice in Nursing?" at https://www.nursingworld.org/content-hub/resources/workplace/evidence-based-practice-in-nursing/.

Instructions

24.1 Identify a project idea at your organization, describe the role of the nurse scientist and bedside scientist in your project, determine what type of project is best for your idea, and conduct a brief literature review on the topic. Record your responses in Table 24.1 and use the literature review template (see Table 24.2).

Project Idea:_____

What is the role of the nurse scientist in the project?

_____

_____

What is the role of the bedside scientist in the project?

_____

_____

TABLE 24.1 NURSE SCIENTIST AND BEDSIDE SCIENTIST ROLES PROJECT

PROJECT TYPE:			
	Definition/Purpose	Rationale	Methodology
Quality improvement			
Evidence-based practice			
Research			

TABLE 24.2 LITERATURE REVIEW TEMPLATE

LITERATURE REVIEW				
Source (Author, Title, Year)	Purpose of Study	Method (including setting and sample)	Key Findings and Implications	Limitations of Study

24.2 Describe the synergistic actions the bedside scientist and the nurse scientist could take to advance your project in a highly reliable organization using Table 24.3 to record your responses.

TABLE 24.3 BEDSIDE SCIENTIST AND NURSE SCIENTIST SYNERGIES

HRO Principles	Definition (Weick & Sutcliffe, 2015)	Nurse Scientist Actions (Kim et al., 2024)	Bedside Scientist Actions (Dunning, 2013; Stutzman et al., 2016)
Sensitivity to operations			
Preoccupation with failure			
Deference to expertise			
Reluctance to simplify			
Commitment to resilience			

CHAPTER 25

ENSURING HIGH RELIABILITY IN ACUTE STROKE TREATMENT

In this chapter, you will learn about how high reliability principles can be used to build a highly reliable team. You will also learn how an acute stroke team used quality tools and change management strategies to implement a critical medication conversion.

Learning Objective

Explore the process of successful identification of failures and planning for change in large and small initiatives.

Learning Activity 25.1: Apply High Reliability Principles to Acute Stroke Treatment

Learning Activity Objectives

25.1 Show several fundamental factors that encourage or act as barriers to successful change in healthcare (*understanding*).

25.2 Apply the methods used in the chapter to a familiar example of a clinical practice change that either went well or did not go well (*applying*).

Preparation

Prior to completion of the learning activity, you should:

- Read Chapter 25.

Instructions

25.1 Identify and discuss a successful change initiative in your organization. What made it possible? Identify and discuss a change initiative in your organization that was *not* successful? What were the items that led to an unsuccessful implementation?

_____

_____

_____

_____

_____

_____

25.2 Identify the items in the chapter that led to a successful implementation. Discuss several of these items and how they might have improved the outcomes in the unsuccessful implementation that you identified above.

_____

_____

_____

_____

_____

_____

PART VIII

TRANSLATION INTO PRACTICE

Learning Objective

Integrate high reliability principles into healthcare practice (*creating*).

Contents

Chapter 26	High Reliability Performance During a Pandemic	90
Chapter 27	Building a High Reliability Head and Neck Operating Room Team	92
Chapter 28	Decreasing Harm From Workplace Violence	96
Chapter 29	Introduction of High Reliability to Frontline Staff: Creating a Virtual Resource Toolkit	99

CHAPTER 26

HIGH RELIABILITY PERFORMANCE DURING A PANDEMIC

In this chapter, you will learn how outbreaks in infectious disease can be anticipated. You will learn about infectious disease outbreak interventions when using the principles of high reliability to achieve a target of zero preventable harm.

Learning Objective

Describe identification and prevention of the spread of infectious diseases.

Learning Activity 26.1: Explore High Reliability Performance During a Pandemic

Learning Activity Objectives

26.1 Explain lessons learned from the COVID-19 pandemic (*understanding*).

26.2 Apply high reliability principles in emergent infectious disease response (*applying*).

Preparation

Prior to completion of the learning activity, you should:

- Read Chapter 26.
- Read "Adapting and Creating Healing Environments: Lessons Nurses Have Learned From the COVID-19 Pandemic" at https://doi.org/10.1016/j.mnl.2021.10.013.

Instructions

26.1 Discuss the potential for the next pandemic, include what was learned from the COVID-19 experience that could be applied to future pandemics and whether we are better prepared.

_____

_____

_____

_____

26.2 Reflect on your healthcare organization's approach to the COVID-19 pandemic. Include the following in your reflection:

- How did the organization prevent panic?
- How did the organization communicate changes in the emergent environment?
- What was successful?
- What was not successful?
- Identify high reliability principles used when creating solutions in the rapidly changing context.

_____

_____

_____

_____

CHAPTER 27

BUILDING A HIGH RELIABILITY HEAD AND NECK OPERATING ROOM TEAM

In this chapter, you will learn about how high reliability principles can be used to build a highly reliable team. You will learn about how an operating room team made the journey to becoming and continuing to be a highly reliable surgical team.

Learning Objective

Explore how to leverage high reliability principles on an interprofessional team to improve patient safety.

Learning Activity 27.1: Apply High Reliability Principles to Solve Team Quality and Safety Challenges

Learning Activity Objectives

27.1 Apply HRO characteristics to design an interprofessional team practice change that improves a quality/safety measure (*applying*).

27.2 Select an interprofessional team quality/safety improvement opportunity where application of high reliability could make a positive impact (*applying*).

27.3 Design a team project plan using the principles of high reliability to improve the interprofessional team quality/safety opportunity (*creating*).

Preparation

Prior to completion of the learning activity, you should:

- Read Chapter 27.
- Identify an interprofessional team quality/safety improvement opportunity that could be affected by team practice changes.
- Read "Nurse Leaders: Transforming Interprofessional Relationships to Bridge Healthcare Quality and Safety" at https://doi.org/10.1016/j.mnl.2021.12.003.

Instructions

27.1 Identify an interprofessional team quality/safety improvement opportunity that could be affected by team practice changes through the use of high reliability principles.

27.2 Using knowledge of high reliability principles, explain which high reliability principles are relevant in solving the problem you identified and why, recording your answers in Table 27.1.

TABLE 27.1 APPLICATION OF HIGH RELIABILITY PRINCIPLES TO AN INTERPROFESSIONAL TEAM QUALITY/SAFETY IMPROVEMENT OPPORTUNITY

Quality/Safety Improvement Need	Principle 1 Preoccupation With Failure	Principle 2 Reluctance to Simplify	Principle 3 Sensitivity to Operations	Principle 4 Commitment to Resilience	Principle 5 Deference to Expertise

continues

TABLE 27.1 APPLICATION OF HIGH RELIABILITY PRINCIPLES TO AN INTERPROFESSIONAL TEAM QUALITY/SAFETY IMPROVEMENT OPPORTUNITY (CONT.)

Quality/Safety Improvement Need	Principle 1 Preoccupation With Failure	Principle 2 Reluctance to Simplify	Principle 3 Sensitivity to Operations	Principle 4 Commitment to Resilience	Principle 5 Deference to Expertise

27.3 Design an interprofessional team project plan using the principles of high reliability to improve the interprofessional team quality/safety opportunity. There are nine sections to complete for this activity (see Figure 27.1).

1. Describe the quality/safety project.
2. Identify the project deliverables.
3. List the baseline measures related to the project.
4. Complete the project plan charter form.
5. List steps or approaches/ideas on how you, as the team leader, would ensure integration of the high reliability principles into the solution(s).
6. Describe any risks or threats to the project.
7. Briefly describe a communication plan for the project.
8. Briefly describe a training plan for the project.
9. Briefly describe how you would evaluate the project's success.

Potential Project Name/Title		Date	
Requested by		Charter Prepared by	

Background & Business Need: State the business problem/issue to solve or what opportunity exists to improve a business function. What is the current state? Narrative background with drivers for the project.

Project Scope Statement: Summarize the purpose and the intent of the project and describe what the customer (or you) envisions will be delivered.

Project Objectives/Deliverables: Outline the high-level objectives for the project. What will exist when the project is complete? Include the benefits of the project, including how the project will benefit the customers or stakeholders.

Boundaries: What will *not* be included in this project?

Assumptions: What assumptions were made when conceiving this project?

External Dependencies: Note any major external (to the project) dependencies the project must rely upon for success, such as specific technologies, third-party vendors, development partners, or other business relationships. Also identify any other related projects or initiatives.

Project Risks: List any known risks for the project that could impact the success of the project or should be considered when planning. Include risk of change management. Does the value of this project ultimately depend on people changing their work or behavior? Identify risks facing this project or organization if the people side of the project is poorly manned.

Key Stakeholders: List the key stakeholders for the project. Stakeholders are individuals, groups, or organizations that are actively involved in a project, are affected by its outcome, or can influence its outcome. Indicate their role or interest in the project. These stakeholders (or representatives) MAY be invited to participate in a project kickoff session but do not necessarily need to be on the project team. Whose day-to-day work will be impacted by raw processes (systems, tools, job roles, organization structure, etc.) as an outcome or deliverable of this project?

Stakeholder/Stakeholder Group	Role in Project or Impacted by This Project

Required Resources: Identify the known resources that management is willing to commit to the project at this time. Human resources includes key individuals, teams, organizations, subcontractors or vendors, and support functions. This is not the place for the detailed team staff roster for individual names. Identify critical skill sets that team members must have. Other resources could include funding, computers, other equipment, physical facilities such as buildings and rooms, hardware devices, software tools, and training. What level of change management involvement is expected for this project? (e.g., separate change management team, change management representation on the core team or individual team).

Requested Timeline/Milestones: Include end and start dates and key milestones.

FIGURE 27.1 Nine-step project plan template.

CHAPTER 28

DECREASING HARM FROM WORKPLACE VIOLENCE

In this chapter, you will learn about workplace violence in healthcare as well as mitigation strategies. You will also learn how application of high reliability principles and "mindful organizing" can improve workplace violence.

Learning Objective

Discuss workplace violence in healthcare experiences and successful mitigation strategies.

Learning Activity 28.1: Discuss Causes, Consequences, and Interventions to Workplace Violence in Healthcare

Learning Activity Objectives

28.1 Explain the impact of workplace violence, causes, and consequences (*understanding*).

28.2 Choose impactful interventions to decrease harm from workplace violence (*applying*).

Preparation

Prior to completion of the learning activity, you should:

- Read Chapter 28
- Read "The Growing Burden of Workplace Violence Against Healthcare Workers: Trends in Prevalence, Risk Factors, Consequences, and Prevention – A Narrative Review" at https://doi.org/10.1016/j.eclinm.2024.102641.

Instructions

28.1 Discuss your personal experience with workplace violence as a healthcare professional. Include the following in the discussion:

- What happened?
- What was your reaction?
- What do you think provoked the violence?
- What resources were available to you to deal with it in the moment or afterward? Were these resources adequate?

_____

_____

_____

_____

_____

_____

28.2 Create a list of interventions found at your place of work or the literature and rate them from 1 (worst) to 5 (best) in their effectiveness to prevent harm from workplace violence.

1. What are the top five interventions that you believe are the most successful in reducing violence and harm from violence in healthcare?

    a.

    b.

    c.

    d.

    e.

2. Can you identify high reliability principles used in the interventions?

    _____
    _____
    _____
    _____
    _____
    _____

CHAPTER 29

INTRODUCTION OF HIGH RELIABILITY TO FRONTLINE STAFF: CREATING A VIRTUAL RESOURCE TOOLKIT

In this chapter, you will learn about how high reliability principles can be used to build a highly reliable team that is foundational in an HRO. You will learn about how building a resource toolkit can foster an environment of high reliability and promote growth within a culture of safety.

Learning Objective

Explore how to leverage high reliability principles on an organization-level interprofessional team to build a resource toolkit to foster a culture of patient safety.

Learning Activity 29.1: Apply High Reliability Principles to Solve Organizational Team Quality and Safety Challenges

Learning Activity Objectives

29.1 Use HRO characteristics to design a healthcare organization interprofessional resource toolkit that promotes a culture of safety (*applying*).

29.2 Select an interprofessional team where application of high reliability could fulfill an organizational strategic initiative of nurturing a culture of high reliability and patient safety (*applying*).

29.3 Design an interprofessional project plan to develop an organizational resource toolkit using high reliability principles to nurture a culture of high reliability and patient safety (*creating*).

Preparation

Prior to completion of the learning activity, you should:

- Read Chapter 29.
- Identify an interprofessional team to apply high reliability to fulfill an organizational strategic initiative.
- Read "Development and Expression of a High-Reliability Organization" at https://doi.org/10.1056/CAT.21.0314.

Instructions

29.1 Identify an organizational culture of safety strategic initiative that could be affected by an interprofessional resource toolkit using high reliability principles.

29.2 Using knowledge of high reliability principles, explain which high reliability principles are relevant in addressing the strategic initiative and why, using Table 29.1 to record your answers.

TABLE 29.1 APPLYING HIGH RELIABILITY PRINCIPLES TO A STRATEGIC INITIATIVE

Strategic Initiative	Principle 1 Preoccupation With Failure	Principle 2 Reluctance to Simplify	Principle 3 Sensitivity to Operations	Principle 4 Commitment to Resilience	Principle 5 Deference to Expertise

CHAPTER 29 INTRODUCTION OF HIGH RELIABILITY TO FRONTLINE STAFF: CREATING A VIRTUAL RESOURCE TOOLKIT

Strategic Initiative	Principle 1 Preoccupation With Failure	Principle 2 Reluctance to Simplify	Principle 3 Sensitivity to Operations	Principle 4 Commitment to Resilience	Principle 5 Deference to Expertise

29.3 Design an interprofessional resource toolkit project plan using the principles of high reliability to meet an organizational culture of safety strategic initiative. There are nine sections to complete this activity (see Figure 29.1):

1. Describe the quality/safety project.
2. Identify the project deliverables.
3. List the baseline measures related to the project.
4. Complete the project plan charter form.
5. List steps or approaches/ideas on how you, as the team leader, would ensure integration of the high reliability principles into the solution(s).
6. Describe any risks or threats to the project.
7. Briefly describe a communication plan for the project.
8. Briefly describe a training plan for the project.
9. Briefly describe how you would evaluate the project's success.

Potential Project Name/Title		Date	
Requested by		Charter Prepared by	

Background & Business Need: State the business problem/issue to solve or what opportunity exists to improve a business function. What is the current state? Narrative background with drivers for the project.

Project Scope Statement: Summarize the purpose and the intent of the project and describe what the customer (or you) envisions will be delivered.

Project Objectives/Deliverables: Outline the high-level objectives for the project. What will exist when the project is complete? Include the benefits of the project, including how the project will benefit the customers or stakeholders.

Boundaries: What will *not* be included in this project?

Assumptions: What assumptions were made when conceiving this project?

External Dependencies: Note any major external (to the project) dependencies the project must rely upon for success, such as specific technologies, third-party vendors, development partners, or other business relationships. Also identify any other related projects or initiatives.

Project Risks: List any known risks for the project that could impact the success of the project or should be considered when planning. Include risk of change management. Does the value of this project ultimately depend on people changing their work or behavior? Identify risks facing this project or organization if the people side of the project is poorly manned.

Key Stakeholders: List the key stakeholders for the project. Stakeholders are individuals, groups, or organizations that are actively involved in a project, are affected by its outcome, or can influence its outcome. Indicate their role or interest in the project. These stakeholders (or representatives) MAY be invited to participate in a project kickoff session but do not necessarily need to be on the project team. Whose day-to-day work will be impacted by raw processes (systems, tools, job roles, organization structure, etc.) as an outcome or deliverable of this project?

Stakeholder/Stakeholder Group	Role in Project or Impacted by This Project

Required Resources: Identify the known resources that management is willing to commit to the project at this time. Human resources includes key individuals, teams, organizations, subcontractors or vendors, and support functions. This is not the place for the detailed team staff roster for individual names. Identify critical skill sets that team members must have. Other resources could include funding, computers, other equipment, physical facilities such as buildings and rooms, hardware devices, software tools, and training. What level of change management involvement is expected for this project? (e.g., separate change management team, change management representation on the core team or individual team).

Requested Timeline/Milestones: Include end and start dates and key milestones.

FIGURE 29.1 Nine-step project plan template.

PART IX

TRANSLATION INTO PRACTICE SUMMATIVE ASSESSMENT

Learning Objective

Examine how high reliability principles are translated into practice.

Contents

Summative Assessment: Translation Into Practice...........104

Supplemental Resources and Readings............................107

SUMMATIVE ASSESSMENT: TRANSLATION INTO PRACTICE

This summative course assessment evaluates your learning at the end of the course. This assessment may be used as a comprehensive measure of your understanding and ability to translate evidence-based practice (EBP), change management, and high reliability principles to practice.

Learning Objective

Examine how high reliability principles are translated into practice.

Summative Assessment Learning Activity: Translate Evidence-Based Practice, Change Management, and High Reliability Principles to Practice

Summative Assessment Learning Activity Objectives

SA.1 Show an EBP model and a change management model (*understanding*).

SA.2 Summarize characteristics of EBP process, change management, and high reliability principles in one of the provided examples (*understanding*).

SA.3 Apply characteristics of EBP process, change management, and high reliability principles to a student-selected clinical practice problem (*applying*).

Preparation

Prior to completion of the learning activity, you should:

- Read chapters within the textbook that describe a process for improvement of interest.

Instructions

SA.1 Show an EBP model and a change management model. Choose one chapter from the book describing a project that led to an improvement. Using selected EBP and change management models, identify steps of the EBP process and change management process described in the chapter. The EBP Worksheet (Appendix A in this workbook) may be useful for you to complete this exercise. Answer the following questions to evaluate the translation-into-practice example:

1. How did the project use data to identify the need for change or define the problem?

   _____

   _____

2. How was literature used to explain the rationale for the intervention?

   _____

   _____

3. Is the intervention based on a theory?

   _____

   _____

4. How did the authors obtain buy-in from stakeholders?

   _____

   _____

5. Was there any evidence of resistance to change?
_____
_____

6. How was resistance to change addressed?
_____
_____

7. How was data collected and analyzed?
_____
_____

8. Was a tool used for data collection?
_____
_____

9. Is there a plan for sustainability?
_____
_____

SA.2 Summarize characteristics and use of high reliability principles within the aforementioned translation-into-practice example. "High Reliability Organizations: A Quick Guide for Frontline Application," Appendix B of this workbook, may be a useful tool to for completing this exercise.

SA.3 Identify a problem from your own practice and integrate EBP steps, change management principles, and high reliability principles to create a sustainable practice change. Create a basic proposal to describe your plan. Include the following:

- Background and significance of the problem
- Problem statement
- Objectives and aims of the project, intervention description
- Methodology
- Proposed intervention
- Setting and participants
- Proposed outcome measures and evaluation
- Data collection plan
- Data analysis plan

Include a description of a tool or method of high reliability.

Include a description of a principle of change management.

SUPPLEMENTAL RESOURCES AND READINGS

PART I

CHAPTER 1

Conklin, T. *Pre-accident investigation podcast*. https://preaccidentpodcast.podbean.com/

Dekker, S. (2025). *What is safety differently?* https://sidneydekker.com/

Kuhlman, J. & Roncska, R. (2024). *High reliability healthcare: Applying the secrets of the nuclear navy to save patient lives*. Ballast Books. http://www.ballastbooks.com/

Myers, G. & Sutcliffe, K. (2022). High reliability organizing in healthcare: still a long way left to go. *BMJ Quality & Safety*, 31, 845-848. https://doi.org/10.1136/bmjqs-2021-014141

Weick, K. E., & Sutcliffe, K. M. (2015). *Managing the unexpected: Sustaining performance in a complex world*. (3rd ed.). Wiley.

CHAPTER 2

Armstrong, G., & Sherwood, G. (2020). Patient safety. In J. F. Giddens (Eds.), *Concepts for nursing practice* (pp. 434–442). Elsevier.

Barnsteiner, J. (2022). Safety. In G. Sherwood & J. Barnsteiner (Eds.), *Quality and safety in nursing: A competency approach to improving outcomes* (pp. 149–170). Wiley-Blackwell.

Reason, J. (2000). Human error: Models and management. *British Medical Journal*, 320(7237), 768–770. https://doi.org/10.1136/bmj.320.7237.768

Sherwood, G. (2022). Driving forces for quality and safety: Changing mindsets to improve healthcare. In G. Sherwood & J. Barnsteiner (Eds.), *Quality and safety in nursing: A competency approach to improving outcomes* (pp. 3–21). Wiley-Blackwell.

CHAPTER 3

Al-Amin, M., Schiaffino, M. K., Park, S., & Harman, J. (2018). Sustained hospital performance on consumer assessment of healthcare providers and system survey measures. What are the determinants? *Foundation of the American College of Healthcare Executives*, 36(1), 15–28. https://doi.org/10.1097/JHM-D-16-00006

Ellenbogen, M. I., Ellenbogen, P. M., Rim, N., & Brotman, D. J. (2022). Characterizing the relationship between hospital Google star ratings, Hospital Consumer Assessment of Healthcare Providers and Systems (HCAHPS) scores, and quality. *Journal of Patient Experience*, 9, 23743735221092604. https://doi.org/10.1177/23743735221092604

Makic, M. B. F., & Granger, B. B. (2019). Deimplementation in clinical practice. What are we waiting for? *AACN Advanced Critical Care*, 30(3), 282–286. https://doi.org/10.4037/aacnacc2019607

Padula, W. V., Lee, K. K. H., & Pronovost, P. J. (2021). Using economic evaluation to illustrate value of care for improving patient safety and quality: Choosing the right method. *Journal of Patient Safety*, 17(6), e568–e574. https://doi.org/10.1097/PTS.0000000000000410

Sutcliffe, K. M. (2023). Building cultures of high reliability: Lessons from the high reliability organization paradigm. *Anesthesiology Clinics*, 41(4), 707–717. https://doi.org/10.1016/j.anclin.2023.03.012

CHAPTER 4

Bellot, J. (2011). Defining and assessing organizational culture. *Nursing Forum*, 46(1), 29–37. https://doi.org/10.1111/j.1744-6198.2010.00207.x

Cartland, J., Green, M., Kamm, D., Halfer, D., Brisk, M. A., & Wheeler, D. (2022). Measuring psychological safety and local learning to enable high reliability organizational change. *BMJ Open Quality*, 11(4), e001757. https://doi.org/10.1136/bmjoq-2021-001757

Edmondson, A. C. (2019). *The fearless organization: Creating psychological safety in the workplace for learning, innovation, and growth*. Wiley.

Gallo, A. (2023, February 15). What is psychological safety? *Harvard Business Review*. https://hbr.org/2023/02/what-is-psychological-safety

Ito, A., Sato, K., Yumoto, Y., Sasaki, M., & Ogata, Y. (2022). A concept analysis of psychological safety: Further understanding for application to health care. *Nursing Open*, 9(1), 467–489. https://doi.org/10.1002/nop2.1086

CHAPTER 5

Edmondson, A. (2019). *The fearless organization: Creating psychological safety in the workplace for learning, innovation, and growth*. Wiley.

Ford, J. L. (2018). Revisiting high-reliability organizing: Obstacles to safety and resilience. *Corporate Communications: An International Journal*, 23(2), 197–211. https://doi.org/10.1108/CCIJ-04-2017-0034

Omidi, L., Karimi, H., Pilbeam, C., Mousavi, S., & Moradi, G. (2023). Exploring the relationships among safety leadership, safety climate, psychological contract of safety, risk perception, safety compliance, and safety outcomes. *Frontiers in Public Health*, 11, 1235214. https://doi.org/10.3389/fpubh.2023.1235214

Weick, K. E., & Sutcliffe, K. M. (2015). *Managing the unexpected: Sustaining performance in a complex world* (3rd ed.). Wiley.

CHAPTER 6

Jack, L. (2021). Advancing health equity, eliminating health disparities, and improving population health. *Preventing Chronic Disease, 18*, 210264. http://dx.doi.org/10.5888/pcd18.210264

Moy, E., Hausmann, L. R., & Clancy, C. M. (2022). From HRO to HERO: making health equity a core system capability. *American Journal of Medical Quality, 37*(1), 81-83. https://doi.org/10.1097/JMQ.0000000000000020

Togioka, B. M., Duvivier D., & Young, E.(2025, January). Diversity and discrimination in health care. *StatPearls*. https://www.ncbi.nlm.nih.gov/books/NBK568721/

World Health Organization. (n.d.). *Health equity*. https://www.who.int/health-topics/health-equity#tab=tab_1

PART II

CHAPTER 7

CMS. (n.d). *Guidance for performing failure mode and effects analysis with performance improvement projects*. https://www.cms.gov/Medicare/Provider-Enrollment-and-Certification/QAPI/Downloads/GuidanceForFMEA.pdf

Pidgeon, N. (2010). Systems thinking, culture of reliability and safety. *Civil Engineering & Environmental Systems, 27*(3), 211–217. https://www.icesi.edu.co/blogs/pslunes122/files/2012/08/Systems-thinking-culture-of-reliability-and-safety1.pdf

CHAPTER 8

Almansour, H. (2024). Barriers preventing the reporting of incidents and near misses among healthcare professionals. *Journal of Health Management, 26*(1), 78–84. https://doi.org/10.1177/09720634231167031

The Joint Commission. (2018). *Developing a reporting culture: Learning from close calls and hazardous conditions*. https://www.jointcommission.org/-/media/tjc/documents/resources/patient-safety-topics/sentinel-event/sea_60_reporting_culture_final.pdf?db=web&hash=5AB072026CAAF4711FCDC343701B0159

Uibu, E., Põlluste, K., Lember, M., & Kangasniemi, M. (2020). Reporting and responding to patient safety incidents based on data from hospitals' reporting systems: A systematic review. *Journal of Hospital Administration, 9*(2), 22-32. https://doi.org/10.5430/jha.v9n2p22

Woo, M. W. J., & Avery, M. J. (2021). Nurses' experiences in voluntary error reporting: An integrative literature review. *International Journal of Nursing Sciences, 8*(4), 453–469. https://doi.org/10.1016/j.ijnss.2021.07.004

PART III

CHAPTER 9

Dekker, S. (2011). *Patient safety: A human factors approach*. CRC Press.

Holden, R. J., Carayon, P., Gurses, A. P., Hoonakker, P., Hundt, A. S., Ozok, A. A., & Rivera-Rodriguez, A. J. (2013). SEIPS 2.0: A human factors framework for studying and improving the work of healthcare professionals and patients. *Ergonomics, 56*(11), 1669–1686. https://doi.org/10.1080/00140139.2013.838643

Marriott, R. D. (2018). Process mapping–The foundation for effective quality improvement. *Current Problems in Pediatric & Adolescent Health Care, 48*(7), 177–181. https://doi.org/10.1016/j.cppeds.2018.08.010

Weaver, B. W., Gannon, P. R., & Mumma, J. M. (2024). Improving patient safety by design: The role of human factors engineering. In C. A. Oster & J. S. Braaten (Eds.), *The nexus between nursing and patient safety* (pp. 241–257). Springer Nature.

CHAPTER 10

Institute for Healthcare Improvement. (n.d.). *RCA²: Improving root cause analyses and actions to prevent harm*. https://www.ihi.org/resources/tools/rca2-improving-root-cause-analyses-and-actions-prevent-harm#:~:text=This%20tool%20describes%20best%20practices%20for%20conducting%20a,actions%20will%20have%20the%20strongest%20effect%20for%20succes

Maternity & Newborn Safety Investigations. (2024). *Why it made sense at the time: Local rationality questions for healthcare investigations*. https://www.mnsi.org.uk/news/local-rationality-questions-for-healthcare-investigations/

National Patient Safety Foundation. (2016). *RCA²: Improving root cause analysis and actions to prevent harm*. https://www.med.unc.edu/ihqi/files/2018/07/RCA2-National-Patient-Safety-Foundation.pdf

Sampson, P., Back, J., & Drage, S. (2021). Systems-based models for investigating patient safety incidents. *BJA Education, 21*(8), 307–313. https://doi.org/10.1016/j.bjae.2021.03.004

CHAPTER 11

Dekker, S. (2013). *Second victim: Error, guilt, trauma, and resilience.* Chapman & Hall/CRC.

Dekker, S. (2018). *Just Culture: Restoring trust and accountability in your organization* (3rd ed.). Chapman & Hall/CRC.

Marx, D. (2009). *Whack-a-mole: The price we pay for expecting perfection.* By Your Side Studios.

Marx, D. (2019). *Reckless homicide at Vanderbilt? A Just Culture analysis.* https://www.linkedin.com/pulse/reckless-homicide-vanderbilt-just-culture-analysis-david-marx/

Ozeke, O., Ozeke, V., Coskun, O., & Budakoglu, I. I. (2019). Second victims in health care: Current perspectives. *Advances in Medical Education & Practice, 10*, 593–603. https://doi.org/10.2147/AMEP.S185912

Restorative Just Culture Checklist. https://safetydifferently.com/restorative-just-culture-checklist/restorativejustculturechecklist-2/

PART IV

CHAPTER 12

Hravnak, M., Pellathy, T., Chen, L., Dubrawski, A., Wertz, A., Clermont, G., & Pinsky, M. R. (2018). A call to alarms: Current state and future directions in the battle against alarm fatigue. *Journal of Electrocardiology, 51*(6S), S44–S48. https://www.ncbi.nlm.nih.gov/pmc/articles/PMC6263784/pdf/nihms-1502834.pdf

Woo, M., & Bacon, O. (2020, March 13). Alarm fatigue. In K. K. Hall, S. Shoemaker-Hunt, L. Hoffman, et al. *Making healthcare safer III: A critical analysis of existing and emerging patient safety practices.* Agency for Healthcare Research and Quality. https://www.ncbi.nlm.nih.gov/books/NBK555522/

CHAPTER 13

Englebright, J. (2019). *Ideal nursing workflows to support the development of information technology solutions.* Sigma Repository. https://www.sigmarepository.org/gen_sub_csm/30/

Fraczkowski, D., Matson, J., & Lopez, K. D. (2020). Nurse workarounds in the electronic health record: An integrative review. *Journal of the American Medical Informatics Association, 27*(7), 1149-1165. https://doi.org/10.1093/jamia/ocaa050

Soong, C., & Shojania, K. G. (2020). Education as a low-value improvement intervention: Often necessary but rarely sufficient. *BMJ Quality & Safety, 29*(5), 353-357. https://doi.org/10.1136/bmjqs-2019-010411

UC-Davis PSNet Editorial Team. (2019). *Human factors engineering.* Agency for Healthcare Research and Quality, US Department of Health and Human Services. https://psnet.ahrq.gov/primer/human-factors-engineering

CHAPTER 14

Goldenhar, L. M., Brady, P. W., Sutcliffe, K. M., & Muething, S. E. (2013). Huddling for high reliability and situation awareness. *BMJ Quality & Safety, 22*(11), 899–906. https://doi.org/10.1136/bmjqs-2012-001467

Merchant, N. B., O'Neal, J., Montoya, A., Cox, G. R., & Murray, J. S. (2023). Creating a process for the implementation of tiered huddles in a Veterans Affairs medical center. *Military Medicine, 188*(5-6), 901–906. https://doi.org/10.1093/milmed/usac073

PART V

CHAPTER 15

Brooks, A., Fitzpatrick, S., & Dunlap, E. (2022). Creating a culture of teamwork through the use of the TeamSTEPPS framework: A review of the literature and considerations for nurse practitioners. *Journal of Leadership Education, 21*(1), 155–162. https://doi.org/10.12806/V21/I1/R11

Edmondson, A. C. (2012). *Teaming: How organizations learn, innovate, and compete in the knowledge economy.* Wiley.

Rosen, M. A., DiazGranados, D., Dietz, A. S., Benishek, L. E., Thompson, D., Pronovost, P. J., & Weaver, S. J. (2018). Teamwork in healthcare: Key discoveries enabling safer, high-quality care. *American Psychologist, 73*(4), 433–450. https://doi.org/10.1037/amp0000298

CHAPTER 16

Agency for Healthcare Research and Quality. (2023, March). *Guide to patient and family engagement in hospital quality and safety.* https://www.ahrq.gov/patient-safety/patients-families/engagingfamilies/index.html

Agency for Clinical Innovation. (2019). *Patient experience and consumer engagement—A guide to build co-design capability*. https://aci.health.nsw.gov.au/data/assets/pdf_file/0013/502240/ACI-Guide-build-codesign-capability.pdf.

McGowan, D., Morley, C., Hansen, E., Shaw, K., & Winzenberg, T. (2024). Experiences of participants in the co-design of a community-based health service for people with high healthcare service use. *BMC Health Services Research*, 24(1), 339. https://doi.org/10.1186/s12913-024-10788-5

Newman, B., Joseph, K., Chauhan, A., Seale, H., Li, J., Manias, E., Walton, M., Mears, S., Jones, B., & Harrison, R. (2021). Do patient engagement interventions work for all patients? A systematic review and realist synthesis of interventions to enhance patient safety. *Health Expectations*, 24(6), 1905–1923. https://doi.org/10.1111/hex.13343

CHAPTER 17

Caporale-Berkowitz, N., & Friedman, S. D. (2018). How peer coaching can make work less lonely. *Harvard Business Review*. https://hbr.org/2018/10/how-peer-coaching-can-make-work-less-lonely

Kotter, J. (1995, March-April). Leading change: why transformation efforts fail. *Harvard Business Review*. https://hbr.org/1995/03/leading-change-why-transformation-efforts-fail-2

Pfeifer, L., Vessey, J., Cazzell, M., Ponte, P. R., & Geyer, D. (2023). Relationships among psychological safety, the principles of high reliability, and safety reporting intentions in pediatric nursing. *Journal of Pediatric Nursing*, 73, 130–136. https://doi.org/10.1016/j.pedn.2023.09.001

PART VI

CHAPTER 18

National Academies of Sciences, Engineering, and Medicine. (2019). *Taking action against clinician burnout: A systems approach to professional well-being*. The National Academies Press. https://doi.org/10.17226/25521

Rushton, C. H. (2023). Transforming moral suffering by cultivating moral resilience and ethical practice. *American Journal of Critical Care*, 32(4), 238–248. https://doi.org/10.4037/ajcc2023207

CHAPTER 19

International Nursing Association for Clinical Simulation and Learning. https://www.inacsl.org/

Lamé, G., & Dixon-Woods, M. (2020). Using clinical simulation to study how to improve quality and safety in healthcare. *BMJ Simulation & Technology Enhanced Learning*, 6(2), 87-94. https://doi.org/10.1136/bmjstel-2018-000370

CHAPTER 20

Granitto, M., Linenfelser, P., Hursey, R., Parsons, M., & Norton, C. (2020). Empowering nurses to activate the rapid response team. *Nursing*, 50(6), 52-57. https://doi.org/10.1097/01.NURSE.0000662356.08413.90

Williams, K-L., Rideout, J., Pritchett-Kelly, J., McDonald, M., Mullins-Richards, M., & Dubrowski, A. (2016, December). Mock code: A code blue scenario requested by and developed for registered nurses. *Cureus*, 8(12), e938. http://doi.org/10.7759/cureus.938

Won, Y. H., & Kang, J. (2022). Development of a comprehensive model for the role of the rapid response team nurse. *Intensive & Critical Care Nursing*, 68, 103136. https://doi.org/10.1016/j.iccn.2021.103136

CHAPTER 21

Black, J. S. (2014). *It starts with one: Changing individuals changes organizations* (3rd ed.). Pearson Education.

Dekker, S. (2017). *Just Culture—Restoring trust and accountability in your organization* (3rd ed.). CRC Press/ Taylor & Francis Group.

Rodriguez, R., Hambley, C., & Wisner, K. (2024). Taking the fear out of peer feedback: A brain-friendly peer feedback program. *Journal of Nursing Administration*, 54(1), 40–46. https://doi.org/10.1097/NNA.0000000000001375

PART VII

CHAPTER 22

Auraaen, A., L. Slawomirski, L., & Klazinga, N. (2018), The economics of patient safety in primary and ambulatory care: Flying blind. *OECD Health Working Papers*, No. 106, OECD Publishing. https://doi.org/10.1787/baf425ad-en

Gaguski, M. E., & Nguyen, H. T. (2016). An interdisciplinary approach to the development and implementation of electronic treatment orders in a medical oncology department. *Clinical Journal of Oncology Nursing, 20*(4), 371–373. https://www.ons.org/articles/interdisciplinary-approach-development-and-implementation-electronic-treatment-orders

Siaki, L., Patrician, P. A., Loan, L. A., Matlock, A.M., Start, R. E., & McCarthy, M. S. (2022). Improving 9.5 million lives: Pilot testing ambulatory care nurse-sensitive quality indicators. *Journal of Nursing Administration, 52*(11), 613–619. https://doi.org/10.1097/NNA.0000000000001218

CHAPTER 23

American Nurses Credentialing Center. (n.d.). *Magnet Model – Creating a Magnet Culture*. https://www.nursingworld.org/organizational-programs/magnet/magnet-model/

McGinnis, J., Aquino-Maneja, E., Geloso, K., Zaragoza, C., Spicer, J., & Kawar, L. N. (2024). Regional transformation: An integrated systems approach to Magnet designation utilizing high-reliability organization implementation strategies. *Journal of Nursing Care Quality, 39*(4), 345-353. https://doi.org/10.1097/NCQ.0000000000000782

Rodríguez-García, M. C., Márquez-Hernández, V. V., Belmonte-García, T., Gutiérrez-Puertas, L., & Granados-Gámez, G. (2020). How Magnet hospital status affects nurses, patients, and organizations: A systematic review. *American Journal of Nursing, 120*(7), 28–38. https://doi.org/10.1097/01.NAJ.0000681648.48249.16

CHAPTER 24

American Nurses Association. (June 1, 2023). *What is evidence-based practice in nursing?* https://www.nursingworld.org/content-hub/resources/workplace/evidence-based-practice-in-nursing/

Associates in Process Improvement. (n.d.). How to improve: Model for improvement. *Institute for Healthcare Improvement*. https://www.ihi.org/resources/how-improve-model-improvement

Kim, H. J., Kawar, L. N., Rondinelli, J., Aquino-Maneja, E. M., McGinnis, J. A., Scruth, E., Torgrimson-Ojerio, B., D'Alfonso, J., Watkins, A. M., & Doulaveris, P. (2024). The role of the nurse scientist and nursing research within a national integrated health care system. *Nursing Administration Quarterly, 48*(3), 237–247. https://doi.org/10.1097/NAQ.0000000000000644

Lai, M.M. (2021). Why nursing research matters. *Journal of Nursing Administration, 51*(5), 235-236. https://doi.org/10.1097/NNA.0000000000001005

Mulkey, M. A. (2021). Engaging bedside nurse in research and quality improvement. *Journal for Nurses in Professional Development, 37*(3), 138–142. https://doi.org/10.1097/NND.0000000000000732

CHAPTER 25

Rosário, M., & Fonseca, A. C. (2022). Incorporating quality improvement projects into stroke care and research. *Stroke, 53*(3), e118–e121. https://doi.org/10.1161/STROKEAHA.121.038204

PART VIII

CHAPTER 26

Benton, D.C., Alexander, M., Fotsch, R., & Livanos, N. (August 12, 2020). Lessons learned and insights gained: A regulatory analysis of the impacts, challenges, and responses to COVID-19. *Online Journal of Issues in Nursing, 25*(3). https://doi.org/10.3912/OJIN.Vol25No03PPT51

Doos, D., Hughes, A. M., Pham, T., Barach, P., Bona, A., Falvo, L., Moore, M., Cooper, Dylan D., & Ahmed, R. (2024). Front-line health care workers' COVID-19 infection contamination risks: A human factors and risk analysis study of personal protective equipment. *American Journal of Medical Quality 39*(1), 4–13. https://doi.org/10.1097/JMQ.0000000000000159

Gregory, D. D., Stichler, J. F., & Zborowsky, T. (2022). Adapting and creating healing environments: lessons nurses have learned from the COVID-19 pandemic. *Nurse Leader, 20*(2), 201-207. https://doi.org/10.1016/j.mnl.2021.10.013

Mumma, J. M., Durso, F. T., Casanova, L. M., Erukunuakpor, K., Kraft, C. S., Ray, S. M., Shane, A. L., Walsh, V. L., Shah, P. Y., Zimring, C., DuBose, J., & Jacob, J. T. (2019). Variability in the duration and thoroughness of hand hygiene. *Clinical Infectious Diseases, 69*(Suppl. 3), S221–S223. https://doi.org/10.1093/cid/ciz612

CHAPTER 27

Guttman, O. T., Lazzara, E. H., Keebler, J. R., Webster, K. L., Gisick, L. M., & Baker, A. L. (2023). Closed-loop communication in interprofessional emergency teams: A cross-sectional observation study on the use of closed-loop communication among anesthesia personnel. *Journal of Patient Safety, 19*(2), 93–99. https://doi.org/10.1097/PTS.0000000000001098

Sanchez, J. A., & Barach, P. R. (2012). High reliability organizations and surgical microsystems: Re-engineering surgical care. *Surgical Clinics of North America, 92*(1), 1–14. https://doi.org/10.1016/j.suc.2011.12.005

Stucky, C. H., Wymer, J. A., & House, S. (2022). Nurse leaders: Transforming interprofessional relationships to bridge healthcare quality and safety. *Nurse Leader, 20*(4), 375-380. https://doi.org/10.1016/j.mnl.2021.12.003

CHAPTER 28

American Society for Health Care Risk Management. (n.d.). *Health care facility workplace violence risk assessment toolkit*. https://www.ashrm.org/resources/workplace_violence

O'Brien, C. J., van Zundert, A. A., & Barach, P. R. (2024). The growing burden of workplace violence against healthcare workers: Trends in prevalence, risk factors, consequences, and prevention–a narrative review. *EClinicalMedicine, 72*. https://doi.org/10.1016/j.eclinm.2024.102641

CHAPTER 29

Heron, L., & Bruk-Lee, V. (2020). When empowered nurses are under stress: Understanding the impact on attitudes and behaviours. *Stress & Health, 36*(2), 147–159. https://doi.org/10.1002/smi.2905

Phillips, R. A., Schwartz, R. L., Sostman, H. D., & Boom, M. L. (2021). Development and expression of a high-reliability organization. *NEJM Catalyst Innovations in Care Delivery, 2*(12). https://doi.org/10.1056/CAT.21.0314

Veazie, S., Peterson, K., & Bourne, D. (2019). *Evidence brief: Implementation of high reliability organization principles*. https://www.hsrd.research.va.gov/publications/esp/high-reliability-org-supplemental.pdf

PART IX

SUMMATIVE ASSESSMENT COURSE ASSESSMENT

Cullen, L., Hanrahan, K., Farrington, M., Tucker, S., & Edmonds, C. (2023). *Evidence-based practice in action: Comprehensive strategies, tools, and tips from the University of Iowa Hospitals and Clinics*, (2nd ed.). Sigma Theta Tau International.

Houser, J., & Oman, K. (Eds.). (2011). *Evidence-based practice: An implementation guide for healthcare organizations*. Jones & Bartlett.

Mazurek-Melnyk, B., & Fineout-Overholt, E. (2022). *Evidence-based practice in nursing & healthcare: A guide to best practice* (5th ed.). Wolters Kluwer.

www.ingramcontent.com/pod-product-compliance
Lightning Source LLC
Chambersburg PA
CBHW082213300426
44117CB00016B/2792